The Midwife's Here!

LINDA FAIRLEY

The Midwife's Here!

The enchanting
true story of one
of Britain's longest-
serving midwives

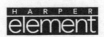

HARPER
element

HarperElement
An imprint of HarperCollins*Publishers*
77–85 Fulham Palace Road,
Hammersmith, London W6 8JB

www.harpercollins.co.uk

and HarperElement are trademarks of
HarperCollins*Publishers* Ltd

Published by HarperElement 2012

3 5 7 9 10 8 6 4 2

Plate section images: p. 1 (bottom) and p. 3 (bottom), courtesy of Manchester Libraries,
Information and Archives, Manchester City Council; p. 2 (top) © D. J. Cunningham, Head
Teacher, Harrytown Catholic High School; p. 6 (top) © Photoshot; p. 6 (bottom) and p. 7
(top and bottom) © *The Times*/NI Syndication

A catalogue record for this book is
available from the British Library

ISBN 978-0-00-744630-8

Printed and bound in Great Britain by
Clays Ltd, St Ives plc

MIX
Paper from
responsible sources
FSC® C007454

FSC™ is a non-profit international organisation established to promote
the responsible management of the world's forests. Products carrying the
FSC label are independently certified to assure consumers that they come
from forests that are managed to meet the social, economic and
ecological needs of present and future generations,
and other controlled sources.

Find out more about HarperCollins and the environment at
www.harpercollins.co.uk/green

For Peter,
who told me I could write this book.
He was so proud of me,
and I know he'd have loved it.

Contents

'Go, and do thou likewise.'

Prologue

'The midwife's here!' Mick Drew exclaimed, nudging his wife Geraldine as I approached her bedside.

Mick gave me a broad smile that was filled with a mixture of gratitude and relief. It was a look I was growing accustomed to seeing on the faces of husbands with expectant wives, and I had learned that the more imminent the birth, the more appreciative and thankful the smile became.

It was early 1971 and Geraldine was about two months away from giving birth, but she was in the highly unusual position of expecting naturally conceived triplets, which no doubt more than trebled her loving husband's concern.

'Flamin 'eck, how long? I'll go round the twist!' Geraldine had balked when I outlined her birth plan a few months earlier, explaining that her multiple pregnancy automatically meant she would be admitted to the antenatal ward in Ashton General Hospital for bed rest when she was seven months pregnant.

'That's the rule, I'm afraid,' I explained, thinking it was unfortunate Geraldine wouldn't benefit from our brand new maternity unit, which wasn't due to open until the end of the year. 'Don't you worry, we'll take good care of you in here and I'm sure you'll enjoy the break.'

Geraldine tittered. 'Well, I suppose rules is rules, though I'm not sure how my old man will take it!'

She and Mick already had three young children, and quite how he was going to cope alone with them while his wife was in hospital was not yet apparent.

'I suppose it'll be good training for him,' Geraldine said cheerfully the last time I saw her at antenatal clinic. 'Seeing as how we're going to end up with six! He'll have to get used to doing his share and keeping an eye on three of 'em.'

I was pleased to see Geraldine had an easy-going nature and was quick to see the funny side of life. She would doubtless need those qualities to cope with a brood that size.

'As for me, I'll just have to get meself a pile of good mags to keep me busy, won't I?' she winked. 'I'm sure I'll cope.'

It hadn't taken Geraldine long to settle herself into the antenatal ward, aided amiably by Mick, who was a round, ruddy-cheeked man who visited often and had such a spring in his step he appeared to bounce down the corridor, flared brown trousers swishing round his ankles.

Every day he wheeled in a little tartan shopping trolley of provisions for his wife and greeted her by planting a huge kiss on both cheeks, and then on the lips. 'One for each baby,' he always beamed before handing Geraldine a packet of sweets or a paper bag containing drinks and magazines.

'How's she doing, Nurse?' he always asked me earnestly. 'Everything as it should be?'

'Yes, everything seems fine,' I reassured him. 'Your wife is doing very well indeed.'

'Terrific!' he grinned. 'She's a coper, my Geraldine, that she is.'

'In't he a smasher, Nurse?' Geraldine would often say after his visits. 'I've got meself a real diamond in Mick, that's for sure.'

I got so used to seeing Geraldine plumped up on a pillow, swathed in a garish purple satin nightgown Mick had bought her at Stockport market, that after just a few weeks it felt as if she'd always been with us. Sometimes she even talked the nurses into letting her help out with the tea trolley, dishing out cuppas to other patients.

'Does me good to stretch me legs,' she'd grin as she waddled round the ward shouting out, 'Two sugars as usual, Mrs Crowe? Best keep your strength up!'

'Evening, Nurse!' she'd always bellow when I turned up for a shift. 'How are you tonight?'

'It's me who should be asking you that,' I'd laugh, marvelling at how much energy Geraldine had in her condition. 'I'll be round later, make sure you're OK.'

When a woman is expecting triplets she is at greater risk of developing high blood pressure, protein in the urine and oedema of the ankles, all of which are complications that can threaten the safety of the mother and baby.

I knew Geraldine wasn't averse to sneaking to the toilets for a cigarette because I often smelled it on her breath, so I was always very particular about checking her blood pressure, in case smoking affected it.

Mick smuggled in the cigarettes, usually hidden in the paper bag he brought beneath a bottle of Vimto, a copy of *Woman's Weekly* and a quarter of pineapple cubes from the corner shop. He tried to be fairly discreet about the cigarettes, but Geraldine didn't really care if she got caught smoking, and often left empty packets and dog ends on the locker beside her bed.

One night as I sat beside Geraldine for a routine blood pressure check, I asked her how she was feeling being stuck in hospital for so long.

'Right as rain,' she chirped. 'To tell you the truth, you were right. I'm enjoying the rest.'

Lowering her voice and staring down at her wedding ring, she added bashfully: 'I'm glad I don't have to face 'im indoors all the time, too.'

'Whatever do you mean?' I asked. 'Mick thinks the world of you, and I thought you said he was a diamond?'

Geraldine leaned her head towards me conspiratorially and fixed her big green eyes on mine. They were glinting with what looked like a mixture of fear and excitement.

'Can you keep a secret, Nurse?' she whispered.

Before I had a chance to answer, Geraldine was mouthing the words: 'They're not his!' As she did so she pointed dramatically to her pregnant belly, which was now so huge it looked fit to burst at any moment.

My eyes felt as if they were bulging out of their sockets, but I tried my best to remain calm and composed in the face of such alarming and unexpected news.

'Well, I don't know what to say,' I blushed. I could feel the colour rising in my cheeks in preparation for her inevitable explanation and confession.

'You see, Nurse, I'm not proud of it, but I went out to a dance in Tarporley and got drunk. I was on those Cinzano and lemonades. Not used to 'em. I had a one-night stand and, trust my luck, I landed up with triplets! Can you believe it?'

She chuckled half-heartedly while I gaped open-mouthed and shook my head.

'No, nor could I, especially when I missed my next period and worked out the dates. Mick had been away, you see, got a big job laying Tarmac on the new motorway in Lancaster. You won't say anything, will ya, Nurse?'

I patted her hand and gave her a big smile. 'Course not,' I said. 'Why would I? Looks like he loves you to bits. I wouldn't dream of interfering. Now come on, get some sleep. Those babies could come any day now you're thirty-five weeks pregnant.'

I was absolutely stunned by Geraldine's revelation, and not altogether certain I'd done the right thing in playing down her infidelity. It wasn't my place to judge her, of course, but now I felt complicit in the deceit and I wished she'd never confided in me. That said, I found it impossible to be cross with Geraldine. She was such a likeable woman, as down to earth as they come. Her secret was safe with me.

The following night I arrived for duty on the labour ward to find an ashen-faced Mick pacing the corridor and dragging urgently on a cigarette, his brow deeply furrowed. For an awful moment I feared he'd found out the terrible truth, but he brightened immediately when he saw me and said: 'It's *very* good to see you, Nurse.'

It seemed Geraldine was in labour, several days earlier than anticipated.

'Look after her, won't you, Nurse?' Mick added, giving me a friendly wink. 'She's the love of my life, you know.'

His words brought a tear to my eye, but it was a happy tear. His sentiments put everything in perspective. He and Geraldine loved each other and they were stuck together like glue. Wasn't that what mattered most? I thought so, and I dearly hoped so.

As Geraldine had been in hospital for practically two months we were well prepared for the triplets' birth. The theatre was ready in case she needed a Caesarean section, but the consultant had decided to give her every opportunity to deliver the babies naturally, as that was the preferred option in the early Seventies, provided there were no complications. We had a team of staff briefed and raring to go, and there had been quite a buzz around the maternity unit for weeks now as we all looked forward to this moment.

I was very proud to have been chosen as one of the three midwives who would each deliver a triplet. It was unusual to have more than one midwife involved, but that was what the doctors had decided on this occasion. I was delighted to have a starring role in the proceedings, and I was also very pleased to have arrived for my shift in good time, while Geraldine was in the first stage, still labouring.

I quickly pinned on my cap, tied on a clean apron and gathered my notes before marching as briskly as my legs could carry me to the delivery room.

Geraldine spotted me the second I walked through the door. 'Glad you're here, Nurse!' she roared between hefty contractions that made her face contort beyond recognition.

Also gathered were two other duty midwives, Jill and Sheila, two trainee doctors I had never met before and two nurses I recognised from theatre and the neonatal unit.

I watched intently as the consultant, Dr Cooper, listened with an ear trumpet for three babies' heartbeats and announced to the room he was extremely pleased to report they all sounded strong and healthy.

My own heart rate was raised at the excitement of the occasion, but I wasn't nervous. Geraldine was a model patient – that's if you discount her frequent, ear-splitting cries of 'Bloody hell!' and 'Flamin' 'eck!'

She gestured for me to take her hand, and each time another contraction came she squeezed so hard I thought she'd cut off my circulation. We spent about two hours going through the same routine of screaming and hand squeezing and, as the labour increased, so too did the volume of Geraldine's cries and the strength of her already vice-like grip.

To help her cope with the pain she sucked on gas and air, which was attached to a big cylinder labelled 'Entonox'. We were ready to give her a shot of the painkiller Pethidine should she require more relief, but in the event her labour progressed so quickly and Geraldine was doing so well, there was no need. At about 11 p.m. the birth began in earnest, with the head of the first of the three babies visible, ready to be delivered.

'I can see baby's head. It's time to push,' I said.

'About bloody time. Aaaaarrrghhhh!' growled Geraldine, before pushing out baby number one beautifully, straight into my hands. It was an absolute joy to see she was a perfect little girl who was so fair she looked as bald as an egg.

As I set about cleaning the screaming baby, who was clearly in no need of resuscitation, I realised Dr Cooper had stepped in to deliver the second baby. He told us it was intent on coming out bottom-first, which wasn't what we'd wanted. Of course, having no scanning equipment in those days and only using our hands to palpate the abdomen and feel the position of the babies, it had been very difficult to gauge accurately how the triplets were lying.

I glanced at my colleague Jill, who had been meant to deliver baby number two. She looked disappointed, but we all knew that a doctor had to deal with a breech birth in these circumstances. Midwives are there to deliver babies under normal conditions, and this was a complication in an already unusual pregnancy.

Somewhere amid Geraldine's now blood-curdling screams and the hushed but firm instructions being issued by Dr Cooper, I heard the words: 'Well done. It's a boy!'

By now baby number three was obviously in a hurry to meet its siblings. 'Cephalic' I heard almost immediately, and breathed a sigh of relief. That meant this one was head first, thank goodness. 'And another girl! Congratulations, Mrs Drew!'

I looked at Geraldine's exhausted face and her eyes met mine. Often during a delivery the mother will seek out one individual for reassurance. Nowadays it is usually the husband, but with Mick still pacing the corridor outside, as expectant dads did back then, Geraldine looked to me in this room full of people.

'Well done,' I whispered. 'You've done it!'

It was only then she allowed a smile to stretch across her face. Despite her brave banter, she had been as apprehensive as the rest of us about this tricky delivery. So much might have gone wrong. Three babies meant three times the potential problems – and some.

'Are they all OK?' Geraldine puffed as I helped clean the babies up and arrange them in three cots around her bed.

'They sound it!' I laughed as the trio struck up a hearty chorus. They were captivating, they really were. Each one was perfect and pink and utterly gorgeous. 'And I can count thirty fingers and thirty toes,' I added, looking adoringly at each one in turn. 'They are wonderful! Shall I get Mick?'

'Yes please,' she nodded proudly.

I have never seen a man look as delighted and besotted as Mick did that day.

'Well, what d'ya reckon?' Geraldine asked as he stepped into the room, his dancing eyes not knowing which cot to peer into first.

'I'm as chuffed as mint balls!' he said, smothering Geraldine with kisses before going up to each cot in turn and cooing over his babies. 'Chuffed as mint balls!'

It was wonderful to witness a show of such pure, unadulterated joy and love. My heart went out to the Drews. They were now responsible for six children under the age of seven. Geraldine had already told me that Mick's wage only just supported them as a family of five, let alone eight. Now they would somehow have to find room for three more little mites in their small semi-detached house. With Geraldine not able to drive and certainly not able to afford a vehicle big enough for her family even if she wanted to, she would have to go everywhere on foot. She would be practically housebound, I realised, with a sudden pang of worry. How would they manage?

Looking at the Drews, who were now holding hands tenderly and gazing at their triplets through dewy eyes, you would never have guessed their world was anything less than perfect. The babies had been delivered safely and each one looked a picture of health. To them, nothing else mattered in that moment, and I was absolutely thrilled for them.

Geraldine and her babies spent ten more days with us. We placed three cots around her bed on the postnatal ward, and at night all three babies were taken to the nursery, where I would often feed one with a bottle while rocking the other two in their cots using my feet.

I felt sad when I finally said goodbye to Geraldine. Despite her smoking and cursing and despite what she had done behind her husband's back, she was a very nice woman who had a heart of gold, and I knew I would miss her. I still felt uneasy about the deceit, of course. I desperately wanted things to work out for the Drew family and I couldn't help worrying about what might happen if Mick ever discovered his wife's guilty secret.

'Daddy, baby Michael looks the spit of you!' one of the young Drew boys had exclaimed during an evening visit. 'Look at his big ears! He has your nose too!'

'What do you think, Nurse?' Mick said, directing a piercing gaze at me, which he held for longer than was comfortable.

'Don't ask me!' I laughed, sounding rather too jolly and wishing myself far away. 'All I know is you're a very lucky man, Mr Drew,' I added hastily as I busied myself writing up notes.

'I know, and my wife's a lucky girl,' he said, giving me one of his twinkling winks and smiling a wide, knowing smile. 'A *very* lucky girl indeed.'

He was a card all right, just like Geraldine. They made a good pair and I hoped they made it, I really did.

It wasn't until I was heading home after my shift that something dawned on me. Maybe Mick was trying to tell me something that night? I wondered if he knew the truth all along, or at least suspected it, yet he loved his wife so much he wasn't going to let it spoil a thing? He was a proud and staunch family man, perhaps so much so he was prepared to keep his wife's secret and raise another man's children. It was possible the only thing he wasn't comfortable with was allowing the midwife to think she knew more than he did himself about his personal life.

'A couple of cards all right,' I chuckled to myself when the pieces of the puzzle fell into place in my mind. 'Good luck to them.'

Preface

To this day, the story of Geraldine Drew and the birth of her triplets remains one of my all-time favourites. It encapsulates the role of a midwife as a professional assistant and confidante, whose ultimate aim is to help women deliver babies safely into the world, whatever the circumstances.

The *Oxford English Dictionary* defines a midwife as 'a nurse (typically a woman) who is trained to assist women in childbirth'. Over the decades, I have learned that there are many, many different ways a midwife can assist a woman in childbirth and, believe you me, plenty of them are not listed in midwifery textbooks!

When I started my nursing training in 1966 at the Manchester Royal Infirmary (MRI) I had no idea what I was letting myself in for, or even that I would become a midwife. I have since delivered more than 2,200 babies and I still tingle with excitement at every birth. Just feeling the warmth of a newborn's head in your hands, that new life, there's honestly nothing like it.

In 2010 I celebrated forty years as a qualified midwife, becoming Britain's longest-serving midwife at the same hospital. Today, I marvel at how much, yet also how very little, has altered over the years. I've witnessed countless changes in the

NHS and in midwifery practices, from the demise of the old Nightingale wards to incredible breakthroughs in pregnancy drugs and IVF. I've seen fashions for routine enemas, bottle-feeding and home births come and go, and I've watched the reluctant shuffle of dads into antenatal classes and delivery suites turn into a stampede.

There have been nine changes of government during my career, so I'm told, but I have never let politics get in the way of delivering babies. I have been very happy sailing along in the great old liner that is the NHS, quietly navigating sea changes in bureaucracy, funding, practices and guidelines. I've never aspired to rise up the ranks and become a manager. Delivering babies and striving to make every pregnant woman feel like the most important pregnant woman in the world is what I do best.

Last year I had the honour of being my daughter's midwife during her pregnancy, and I am now a very proud grand-mother. Baby Joel was born prematurely in July 2011 as I was working on this book and also mourning the death of my third husband, Peter.

So much has happened over the years that I could not fit my memoirs into one volume, and this book concentrates on the early years of my career in the late Sixties and early Seventies. That means the story of Joel's nerve-racking birth, along with so many others, will have to wait.

As you read this first instalment, I will keep laughing and crying, remembering and writing.

Chapter One

'It feels like we're in the Army!'

'My job is to make nice young ladies of you all,' Sister Mary Francis proclaimed. She was the headmistress at the strict Harrytown High School I attended in Romiley, Cheshire, and this was a phrase I heard countless times from the age of seven.

The private, all-girls convent school was very highly regarded and, like many of my peers, I came from a comfortable, middle-class family. It was expected that we 'young ladies' would enter suitably respectable employment at the age of eighteen, which I gathered meant choosing between working in a bank, going into teaching or becoming a nurse.

I was seventeen years old when I was summoned to Sister Mary Francis's imposing dark-wood office and asked the question: 'Well, Linda, what do you propose to do next?' Before I could answer, she tilted her head forward to peer at me over her small, round reading glasses and said gravely: 'You are indeed a fine young lady, despite the one minor indiscretion we have thankfully overcome. I trust you have chosen wisely.'

'I'm thinking of going into nursing,' I replied meekly, blushing at her reference to my 'indiscretion'. She meant the time I was caught breaking a cardinal rule and talking to boys on the bus. This had been seen as such a scandalous breach of conduct that a letter was sent home to my parents, warning of severe consequences should I ever compromise my reputation in such a way again.

'Nursing is a good choice for you,' Sister Mary Francis deemed. 'But only the best will do for my girls. I want you to apply to the Manchester Royal Infirmary. It is a teaching hospital, and the most prestigious in the region. Please promise me, Linda, that you will always work hard for your living.'

I nodded obediently, grateful that Sister Mary Francis had not probed any deeper, as I had just three rather fragile reasons behind this big decision.

Number one: my best friend Sue Smith from school had an older sister called Wendy who was a nurse. She was always smiling when she told us tales about her job, and I thought she looked wonderful in her smart uniform. I admired her, and I wanted a uniform like hers.

Number two: my mum always said I was a caring person, telling me that I'd insisted on looking after my teddy bear right up to the age of eleven. I thought I'd be good at tucking patients into bed and giving them tea and sympathy.

Number three: I didn't want to work in a bank and I didn't want to teach. My parents never wanted me to work for the family business, even though their bakery shop near our home in Stalybridge was very successful. It was hard graft being self-employed, Mum always said. She wanted better for me.

Nursing it was to be, and that is how I found myself standing before Miss Morgan, Matron of the Manchester Royal Infirmary, in September 1966.

'You must see me as your other mother!' she boomed. I was eighteen years old and I had just started my three-year training course at the MRI, which was situated on Oxford Road, a mile and a half outside the city centre.

Though I knew next to nothing about nursing I had quickly cottoned on to one very important fact: Matron was like God, and her word was Gospel.

'I want you to be able to talk to me at all times,' Miss Morgan instructed forcefully, her extremely large bust somehow expanding further still as she snorted in her next breath. 'You are *my* girls!'

I looked at her in horror. She seemed completely unapproachable and absolutely nothing like my own mother. My mum was so gentle-natured she practically had kindness dripping from her pores. Miss Morgan was a bulldozer in a bra by comparison. Her voice penetrated my eardrums with considerable force, and her facial expressions were as stiff as the large, starched white frill cap that was clamped on her head.

I nervously glanced from left to right to see how the other new girls in my group were reacting. There were thirty-six teenage girls in my intake, and we were divided into groups of six. As my name then was Linda Lawton, I'd been placed with two other student nurses whose surnames began with the letter L, as well as with three whose surnames began with M and P.

I took some small comfort from the fact Nessa Lawrence, Anne Lindsey, Jo Maudsley, Linda Mochri and Janice Price all looked as startled as I felt.

'You will be taken down shortly to be measured for your new uniforms,' Matron went on, forcing a rather frosty smile to her lips. I imagined her heart was probably in the right place, but she seemed oblivious to the fact she'd turned us into a group of baby rabbits caught in the glaring headlights that were her wide, all-seeing eyes.

'Be warned, girls, that if I catch any of you shortening your uniform I will unpick the hem myself forthwith and restore it to its correct length, which is past your knee, on the calf.

'Hair is to be clean and neat and worn completely off the collar, stocking seams are to be poker straight, and make-up and jewellery are strictly forbidden. Strictly forbidden!

'You will require two pairs of brown lace-up shoes which are to shine like glass every day. Cleanliness is next to godliness, never forget that, girls!'

We listened attentively, scarcely daring to breathe lest we incur Matron's wrath.

'Furthermore,' she went on, 'I will not tolerate lateness, sloppiness or untidiness of any nature and I expect best behaviour at all times.

'Good luck, girls,' she added briskly, smoothing her hands down the front of her exceptionally well-pressed grey uniform. 'Don't forget you must come and talk to me at once about any concerns you may have. I am here to help you.'

Miss Morgan was clearly exempt from the make-up ban as she had thickly painted red lips, which she now stretched into the shape of a wide smile. Despite this she still managed to look incredibly intimidating as she waved us out of her office and instructed us to follow a grey-haired home sister down to the uniform store, a visit she hoped we would all '*thoroughly* enjoy'. Miss Morgan sounded sincere, but in that moment I felt a pang of real fear and homesickness.

The home sisters were typically older, unmarried sisters who had retired from working on the wards but ran the nurses' home, and usually lived in. This one was glaring at us impatiently, which did nothing to ease my anxiety.

Dad had driven me in to Manchester and dropped me off earlier that day, and my small suitcase was still unopened. I'd felt as if I was going on an exciting adventure as we pulled up outside the grand red-brick façade of the enormous teaching hospital. It was opposite the sprawling university campus on Oxford Road, and I felt honoured to be entering the heart of such a vibrant, progressive community.

As I waved Dad off and joined the other eager-looking student nurses gathered in reception, I was buzzing with anticipation. I was actually going to be a nurse, and not just any nurse: I was going to be an MRI nurse!

Now, however, reality was rapidly starting to dawn. I felt lost and abandoned in this unfamiliar environment, with the imposing Miss Morgan thrust upon me as my 'other mother'. Home was less than ten miles away, just a half-hour car ride east of Manchester. It was tantalisingly close, which only made me long for it all the more.

I'd been on just one previous visit to the MRI several months earlier after my letter of application, vetted and approved by Sister Mary Francis, was swiftly accepted. It was June 1966 when I was invited on a whistle-stop tour of the hospital, and when I met some of the other student nurses for the very first time.

Now, I realised, I had scarcely taken anything in. At the time I was preoccupied with finishing my A-levels and going on a summer holiday with my best friend Sue from school. We'd been invited to Beirut in the August, where my brother John, who was ten years older than me, worked as a journalist. It was a very safe and beautiful place to visit in 1966, and we were looking forward to exploring it, then spending two weeks sunning ourselves in Turkey afterwards.

When I got back from that first visit, my boyfriend Graham, who I'd been seeing for about a year, asked, 'What was it like at the MRI?'

'Well, there was nothing I disliked,' I replied cheerfully. 'I think I'll like it,' I added naïvely. 'Shall we go to the cinema in Manchester tonight? I have to get used to the city before I live there!'

How I was ruing my blasé attitude. I was pitifully unprepared for my new life. I had absolutely no clue what I was letting myself in for and I had foolishly committed myself to the MRI for three long years of my life. That's how long it took to qualify as a State Registered Nurse (SRN). Three whole years! I'd be twenty-one before I finished my training. It felt like a lifetime.

Walking along the windowless corridors on the first day of training, I felt like an inmate. Miss Morgan had said we would be 'taken down' to the uniform store, but I felt as if I was being taken down quite literally, to be incarcerated. There was no way out, and I saw nothing to cheer me up.

Plain, white walls were pitted with monochrome signs I didn't understand. Metal trolleys were pushed by porters with faces as dull as cobbles. The hard floors appeared to have been scrubbed clean of any hint of colour. It was just like watching a boring old documentary on television, where everything was a grim shade of black and white.

Big doors loomed everywhere, swinging heavily on their hinges in the wake of white coats and pale green uniforms, which disappeared into goodness knows where. The world beyond the doors was, as yet, a complete mystery to me. The wards and clinics and theatres filled me with a mixture of curiosity and fear. I was in uncharted territory. That's how the hospital seemed to me as I proceeded towards the uniform store with the other girls, marching rigidly on the left-hand side of the corridor, as instructed.

Turning a corner, I felt a gentle dig in the back of my ribs and whipped my head round to see that one of the girls in my group, Linda Mochri, was giving me a cheeky smile.

'What d'ya think of our second Ma, hey Linda?' she asked in a friendly Scottish brogue.

I sniggered and whispered behind my hand: 'I don't think I'd like to fall out with her!'

Linda screwed up her eyes and gave a little chuckle. 'I might have to risk it if the uniform makes me look like a nun!' she joked.

We continued in silence, fearful of receiving a ticking off from the home sister who was accompanying us, but thanks to Linda I felt ever so slightly less alone. We were all in the same boat, weren't we? We 'newbies' would stick together and have a laugh and make the best of it, wouldn't we?

Being measured for my uniform made me imagine I was joining the Army instead of the nursing profession. We had to stand in a stiff line like soldiers as we each took it in turns to have the tape measure wrapped around our bust, waist and hips. All the while we listened earnestly to a string of orders and instructions from the home sister.

'You must wear your uniform at all times, even in school, though you must remove your apron during lessons.

'You will each be provided with three brand new dresses and ten aprons. It is your duty to take good care of your clothing and to take pride in your appearance at all times.

'As you are aware, the uniform consists of a light green dress with detachable white cuffs and collars and a white cap, which must be clean and stiffly starched at all times.

'You will leave your dirty clothes in your named laundry bag outside your room once a week, and they will be taken away and laundered. It is your duty to collect your clean laundry from the uniform collection point.

'You will be shown how to fold your hats correctly, don't fret. You will soon be experts in the art. If you have not already done so you must purchase two pairs of brown lace-up shoes, and your stockings must be brown and seamed. Matron likes seams to be perfectly straight, and be aware she will check up on you without warning.'

As the day went on we were bombarded with more and more information, and my head began to ache. We were shown the stark schoolroom, which contained dark-wood desks, a full-sized skeleton and a dusty blackboard. Our daily routine was to begin at 8 a.m. prompt for lectures with Mr Tate, to whom we were briefly introduced. I scarcely took in a word he said because I was too busy taking in his demeanour. He had huge lips, wore a terrible green knitted tie and ill-fitting glasses, and had the worst comb-over you could ever imagine, with skinny strands of greying hair stretched desperately across his bald scalp. Odd, I thought. A very odd-looking man indeed.

We would spend our first eight-week 'block' based in the schoolroom, and classes would be punctuated with tours of the fourteen wards in the 400-bed hospital. I didn't even know what some of the names of the wards meant, such as endocrinology and thoracic, let alone how to navigate my way through the three-floored maze to find them.

That first evening I sat on my single bed at the nurse's home with all my day's thoughts and fears clattering around inside my aching head. As students we all had to live in the nurses' quarters adjacent to the hospital; there was no choice in the matter. The money for our board was taken out of our student wages before we received them, leaving us first years with £27 a month – not a bad sum to live on, I supposed.

This was the first time I had been alone all day, and I gulped as I sat on the unfamiliar bed, trying to absorb the huge step I was taking. I surveyed my new bedroom warily and felt my throat tighten. It was a large room with a wooden floor and a big fitted wardrobe, which was painted the same drab, off-white colour as the bare walls and had three hefty drawers underneath. I got up and tried to pull one of the drawers open, but found the task almost impossible. Puffing and panting, I eventually managed to heave the drawer free, feeling like a feeble little bird struggling to build a nest. I wanted to cry.

There was a stark white ceramic sink in one corner and a small dressing table with a chair in the other. My bed had two grey woollen blankets, and a starched counterpane lay across the top. I plumped my pillow and it felt stiff and scratchy to the touch, which made me even more miserable. To make myself feel better I took my John Lennon poster from my suitcase and stuck it on the wall above my bed. I knew it was against the rules to decorate the walls but I couldn't really see what harm it could do, and I made a mental note to be careful not to damage the paint when I took it down in the future.

'New linen will be left outside your door once a fortnight,' the home sister had instructed. 'You must strip your bed and leave your dirty laundry outside your door, in your laundry bag.'

She'd given us a brisk guided tour of the nurses' accommodation earlier. 'There are wooden blocks fitted to the inside of all of the windows,' she told us in a matter-of-fact tone. 'This is to stop intruders getting in.'

Sitting on my bed that evening, I looked over at the one small rain-smeared window and felt a film of tears mask my eyes. I was used to living in relative luxury, sheltered at my private convent school and cosseted by my parents in our comfortable suburban home. This was the first time in my whole life I had felt vulnerable – afraid, even. I'd imagined that after spending a month abroad in the summer I'd be absolutely fine living in Manchester. I was less than ten miles from home, but everything here seemed so alien to me.

Sue and I had stayed at my brother's apartment in Beirut for two fun-filled weeks. He worked for United Press International and had a wonderful lifestyle. A cleaner came in every morning while Sue and I sunned ourselves by the pool. Afterwards we met John for lunch at the plush St George's Hotel, and in the evenings he took us to fancy parties. I remembered how he smiled when we asked for Ovaltine at bedtime on our first night. 'Why don't you try a gin and tonic instead?' he suggested. We did, and we never stopped giggling for the whole holiday.

Sue and I both felt so grown-up. We booked ourselves on a three-day excursion to Jerusalem, where I bought a beautiful leather-bound bible, and then we spent two weeks holidaying in Turkey with John's Turkish wife Nevim, who looked after us really well. I was an independent woman of the world – or so I thought.

There was a rap on my door that made me jump. 'Can I come in?' a lovely Scottish voice sang, and I shot up gratefully and unlatched the door.

It knew it was Linda Mochri, and her voice instantly made my tears evaporate.

'Of course you can!' I said, and when I opened the door I was delighted to see she had Nessa, Anne, Jo and Janice in tow.

'Your room's the biggest, you lucky thing!' Linda said as she lit a Marlboro cigarette and sat cross-legged on the end of my bed. The other girls filed in and found themselves a place to sit. Nessa was last through the door and she settled on the scratched wooden floor, folding her enviably long legs beneath her.

Janice also lit a cigarette, which she pulled from a fashionable lacquered case that covered her pack of twenty. She looked confident to the point of cockiness as she took a long drag.

'How are you all settling in, then?' she asked, after blowing out a plume of smoke. She looked at each of us in turn.

'Feels like we're in the Army!' Linda snorted. 'Curfew at 11 p.m., girls!' she said, mimicking the home sister's briefing from earlier in the day. 'Any nurses not home by 11 p.m. will have Matron to deal with and will lose the right to request a late pass! Late passes allow you to be home by midnight – but be warned, you have to earn them, girls!'

We fell about laughing and, with the ice broken, we began to gently pick over the long day we'd had.

'What do you think of our tutor?' Anne asked with a mischievous glint in her eye. Anne was quite plump, with one of those smiley, rosy faces larger girls often have.

We all chipped in with our views on Mr Tate, who for the first two months would teach us anatomy, physiology and basic nursing techniques in the schoolroom. After that he would continue to teach us between our practical training and placements on the wards.

'He's the strangest-looking man I've ever seen,' I volunteered with a shy giggle.

This was no exaggeration. Everyone admitted they had been taken aback at his appearance, particularly his precarious-looking comb-over.

'I dread to think what he looks like when the wind blows,' chuckled Jo.

She and Janice were two of a kind, I thought. Both exuded self-confidence, while Linda and Anne were definitely the jokers in the pack. Nessa seemed more like me. She was softly spoken and came from Cheadle, not too far from where I grew up. We were the only two who didn't smoke, and when Nessa contributed something to the conversation it usually struck a chord with me.

'Is it just me or does anyone else think the blocks on the windows are a bit alarming?' she ventured.

'I hate them!' I admitted. 'It makes me think a mad man is going to break in at any moment.'

'Will you listen to yerself!' Linda mocked gently. 'We're holed up here like prison inmates. I reckon the blocks are there to stop us escaping rather than to stop men breaking in!'

We all laughed again.

'What shall we dissect next?' Anne asked.

'Bathrooms!' Jo and Janice chimed in unison, and we all bemoaned the fact we had one bath and toilet to share between twelve of us.

The nurses' quarters were shaped like a letter 'H' and my new-found friends and I were grouped together down one leg of the 'H'. It was pot-luck that I got the biggest room. We were all allocated a number and I happened to be student nurse number six, which meant I was allocated the sixth room on the corridor.

'It's certainly not what I'm used to,' Anne said wistfully, and we shared snippets of our lives back home.

With the exception of Linda Mochri we had all grown up in the region. Linda's family had relocated from Scotland because her mother was ill with cancer, and the best treatment was available to her in the North West of England. Apart from that, we seemed to have a fair amount in common, all having come from good schools and supportive families. I learned that Linda, Jo and Janice had long-term boyfriends like me, but Nessa and Anne did not.

'This is certainly a far cry from what *any* of us are used to,' Janice declared, wrinkling up her nose.

I couldn't have agreed more. As a child I moved house frequently, always to somewhere bigger and better as Lawton's Confectioners went from strength to strength. My parents sold teacakes, puff pastries, parkin, pies, bread and apple tarts from their double-fronted shop on the High Street in Stalybridge, all hand-made in the bake-house by my father, John.

He was a gentleman who 'never wanted to be on the front row', as my mother Lillian often said. That was absolutely true. You couldn't have met a kinder or more unassuming man, and he never once so much as raised his voice to me. My mother wore the trousers in their relationship and was also the one who controlled the business, but that didn't stop her being a very kind and caring mum.

My brother John and I wanted for absolutely nothing. The fine career in journalism he'd carved out for himself made both my parents very proud and the two of us were the apples of our parents' eyes, in our own distinct ways.

I shared a little bit about my family background with the other girls, and also told them about Graham, who I'd been going out with for about a year.

'I love dancing and we met at the Palais in Ashton last year when I went to a dance with my old school friend Sue,' I told them. 'He works as a car salesman and drives a little blue bubble car.'

'Lucky you! Is he good-looking?' Janice asked cheekily.

'Well, I think so,' I blushed. 'He's got blond hair and blue eyes and wears very nice clothes.'

'Ooooh!' Anne chucked. 'I'm jealous!'

'Come on!' Jo said, sparing me any further interrogation as she stood up and stubbed out her cigarette in my sink, having failed to locate an ashtray. 'We've got an early start tomorrow.' All the other girls took the cue and shuffled to the door.

As I bid them goodnight and got myself ready for bed I couldn't help thinking about my bedroom at home with its soft cotton sheets, plush wool carpet and pretty pictures hung against the stylish floral wallpaper I'd been allowed to pick out from the chic Arighi Bianchi store in Macclesfield. I longed to be back in my bed at home, and for my father to knock gently on my door to wake me up in the morning, as he always did. But then, I thought to myself, what would I do all day?

Here I felt terribly homesick despite the girls' comforting chitchat, but I realised I also felt very much alive and stimulated. My head was filled with hundreds of questions about what tomorrow would bring, and my emotions were on red alert. This experience was unsettling, but it was undeniably exciting too.

It had been an exhausting day, and if my tiredness hadn't knocked me out I'm pretty sure the thick clouds of smoke the girls left behind in my room would have done. I had one of Graham's handkerchiefs, which smelled of his Brut aftershave, and I placed it on my scratchy pillowcase for comfort, and to block out the smell of smoke. I didn't stir until my alarm clock rang at 7.15 a.m., heralding my first full day as a student nurse.

Chapter Two

'I really am becoming an MRI nurse!'

'A patient will not die if you forget to take their blood pressure,' Sister Craddock pealed in her rich Welsh accent as she escorted us from the schoolroom, 'but dirty floors breed bacteria, and bacteria kill.'

Sister Craddock had very curly red hair and a face dotted all over with freckles. Her figure was as round and curvy as her tightly sprung ringlets, and I was as captivated by her appearance as I was by her staunch philosophy on hygiene.

We'd spent the morning studying anatomy with Mr Tate, and my head was brimming with medical facts. I'd enjoyed the lessons and found them easy to follow, because I'd studied chemistry and biology for my A-levels. I pictured myself using my new knowledge, hopefully in the not-too-distant future, to help me bandage a wrist or give a patient an injection. The thought was nerve-racking yet exhilarating.

'Cleanliness is next to godliness,' Sister Craddock chimed, echoing Miss Morgan's words on our very first day here. Spinning on her tightly laced brogues, she looked each of us in the eye one by one as she warned very seriously: 'As a nurse, it is imperative never, ever to forget that.'

This was clearly very important at the MRI. We were student nurses, not cleaners, but I figured I'd better listen as attentively to Sister Craddock as I did to Mr Tate. 'Cleanliness is next to godliness.' I let the phrase settle in my head, wondering what Sister Mary Francis would make of it. In all my years at my convent school I had heard hundreds, if not thousands, of references to 'godliness' but I did not recall that particular phrase. However, I had a pretty good idea I'd be remembering it regularly from now on.

Sister Craddock led a small group of us down several corridors and towards one of the urology wards, continuing to lecture us about hygiene.

'What doesn't kill you makes you stronger,' she said, and I wondered what she could mean by that. Were the cleaning fluids dangerous? What could possibly threaten us here in the hospital? I was getting used to her loud, melodic voice now and my mind was wandering.

As we approached the ward a sudden, silly image flashed into my head. I imagined Sister Craddock stepping up on stage and belting out the song 'Goldfinger'. Shirley Bassey was Welsh, wasn't she? Sister Craddock didn't look anything like Shirley Bassey but she certainly sounded like her. I could just picture her singing her heart out, flinging her arms wide at her grand finale, then afterwards pointing at the audience triumphantly and declaring: 'What doesn't kill you makes you stronger, ladies and gentlemen ...'

'Cleanliness is of the utmost importance on the wards, and to maintain our high standards is *essential*.' Sister Craddock's stern words hauled me back into the moment. Images of sequins and stage lights were extinguished in a flash, replaced by thoughts of dusting cloths, mops, buckets and disinfectant. I listened earnestly.

'We have Nightingale wards here, girls, and if she were alive I would want Florence Nightingale herself to be proud of the cleanliness of them.'

I knew the large, open-plan wards were named after Florence Nightingale because she pioneered their design, but if I'm perfectly honest that was as much as I knew about them, despite their famous namesake. I was curious to find out more.

Sister Craddock pushed her soft bulk through a set of double swing doors, giving us our first glimpse of 'her' ward. The smell of cleaning fluid made my nostrils tingle as I stepped into this new territory. 'Follow me, girls,' she instructed. 'I will give you a brief tour of the ward. Please be respectful of patients. No talking. I will do the talking.'

We stood in the first section of the ward, which Sister Craddock explained had a kitchen and a double side room to the left, and sister's office, linen cupboards and two single side rooms to the right, which we were not invited to enter. Before us stood another set of swing doors, which led into the main part of the ward. We filed gingerly through, eyes and ears wide open.

Twelve beds lined each side of the vast ward, all occupied by ladies in varying stages of sleep who were swathed in flannelette nightgowns and knitted bed jackets. Most looked cosily middle-aged and some wore hairnets and sucked their gums as they surveyed us curiously but courteously.

There was something slightly surreal about the scene that I couldn't quite put my finger on. One or two women were a bit younger and more fashionable than the others, with floral-print nightgowns and bobbed hair, yet there was an unmistakable correlation between them all.

Down the middle of the ward stood the night sister's table, covered in green baize and with a large lamp hanging above it. At night, we were informed, a green cloth was placed over the lamp to create an air of calm and promote restful sleep. Beyond it, but also in the centre section of the ward, was a store cupboard plus a metal trolley housing a sterilising unit, and finally the patient's long wooden dining table.

A sluice room, toilets and a bathroom were situated in the far right-hand corner of the ward, behind bed thirteen. Under the windows at the very back of the ward there was a small television, a few Draylon-covered armchairs and a low coffee table with a neat pile of women's magazines on it. There was also a round, black ashtray, which had a cover. I'd seen one like it before and knew that when you pressed the button on top the ash would spin cleanly out of sight.

Sister Craddock's voice sang on as I took in the scene. 'There are twenty-eight beds in all; four in the side rooms and twenty-four in the main ward. Each ward is run by one sister, six to eight staff nurses and between ten and sixteen student nurses working around the clock. Shifts run from 7 a.m. to 5 p.m., 1.30 p.m. to 9 p.m. and 9 p.m. to 7.30 a.m. Jobs are allocated at each shift change and routines must be strictly adhered to.'

As Sister Craddock spoke, a penny slowly dropped for me. I looked at the twelve beds lined up along each white-painted wall and realised how perfectly arranged they were.

'The ward has to be clean, neat and tidy at all times,' the Welsh voice continued. 'Patients are washed and have their beds changed every day. Bedding must be fitted exactly the same way each day, with enveloped corners on bottom sheets, pillowcase ends facing away from the doors and perfectly folded counterpanes on top of the blankets. You will receive precise instruction in bed-making procedures in due course. Please remember always to pull the top sheet up a little to make room for the toes, and to leave the counterpanes hanging at the sides, for neatness. The wheels of the bed must all point in the same direction, and nothing is to be left lying around on the tops of the lockers.'

That was it. The immaculate presentation of the beds and furniture was what made the ward appear slightly surreal. I had never seen such a well-ordered room in my life before, and I marvelled at how a ward full of sick women in a mish-mash of nighties and hair nets could look so methodically well ordered.

The crisp cotton counterpanes were all pale green to match the curtains that could be pulled around each bed. Every bedside locker had a little white bag taped to it for rubbish, leaving the top clear for a jug of fresh drinking water and a glass. Some patients had a vase of flowers on their locker-top or one or two get well cards.

'Only one bunch of flowers is permitted per patient,' Sister Craddock cautioned, 'and it must be removed to the bathroom at night.'

We nodded in unison. Rudimentary biology told me this had something to do with plants releasing carbon dioxide into the atmosphere at night.

'Smoking is permitted on the ward but not encouraged.' We nodded in agreement again. This seemed perfectly reasonable.

'Orderlies damp dust every surface in the ward daily: windowsills, lockers, bed frames and furniture. Domestics clean the floors, toilets, bathroom, kitchen and sister's office, and twice a week they pull out the beds and clean behind them, *thoroughly*.

'As a student nurse you will be expected to attend to the general good hygiene of the patients and help maintain the high standards of cleanliness required on the wards. It has been said that you could eat your dinner off the floor of my ward, and that is how it must always be. Please always ensure that even the wheels of the bed are gleaming and, of course, neatly aligned after cleaning. If ever you find yourself with a spare moment, use it to pick up a cloth and damp dust. There is always a surface to be dusted and cleaned, and there is no room here at the MRI for nurses who are slothful or slipshod.'

I watched a sympathetic-looking nurse plump up an elderly patient's pillow and fill her glass with fresh water. The patient smiled at the nurse as if she was an angel, and the nurse smiled back, explaining courteously that it was time for the patient's daily injection. The nurse must have been a third year, as she had three stripes of white bias binding on the sleeve of her uniform.

I looked at her in awe and admiration, noting that her bedside manner was as impeccable as her uniform. I wanted to make patients feel better too. I wanted to give them their medicine along with a warm smile. I wanted to be just like that nurse.

A few days later I went to the uniform store with Linda and Nessa, where we were each handed a hessian laundry sack with our names printed neatly across the top in black marker pen. Inside we found our brand new uniforms: three light green dresses made of a sturdy cotton which felt stiff, like new denim, plus ten aprons, three detachable collars and cuffs and a rectangle of white cotton. Sister Craddock deftly demonstrated how to craft the cotton into a perfect cap.

The three of us exchanged knowing glances as we signed for our uniforms and acknowledged the rigid rules about laundering them. This was the moment we'd been looking forward to above all else.

'I can't wait to try this on,' Nessa whispered shyly to me.

'Me too,' I said. 'I hate walking around the hospital in mufti.'

Linda chuckled. 'Hark at you!' she teased. 'A week ago you didn't even know what the word meant!'

My cheeks reddened. It was true. I'd had no idea nurses used the term 'mufti' when referring to their 'civvies' or ordinary clothes, but I'd heard it so many times since our arrival that it had slipped into my vocabulary without me even realising.

'We're going to be proper nurses now,' I grinned, picking up my prized laundry bag. 'We have to use the correct language!'

We carried our uniforms back to the nurses' home with some ceremony, and all agreed to meet in my room for a 'fashion parade' before tea.

My mum had taken me on a shopping trip to Manchester a few weeks earlier and bought me two pairs of comfortable brown lace-up brogues in Freeman Hardy Willis. We had tea and scones with jam and cream in Kendals department store before visiting its grand lingerie section, where she bought me two suspender belts with metal clasps and seven pairs of brown, 30-denier Pretty Polly seamed stockings.

Now I took the underwear out of its tissue wrappers for the first time, and set about clipping, buttoning and lacing myself into my complete nurse's uniform. I was beside myself with excitement as I pulled on my dress and attached its crisp white cuffs and collar, which had to be buttoned onto the dress. Next I used half a dozen brand new kirby grips to pin my neatly folded cap on top of my hair, which I had scraped back off my face and fixed in a tight bun using several brown elastic bands.

Finally, I placed my stiff white apron over my dress. It was huge! The lower part amply covered my wide skirt, which reached almost halfway down my calves, and the two enormous front flaps that pulled up and over each shoulder came so high they covered half of my neck. The wide straps had to cross over my shoulderblades before being brought back round and attached with a thick safety pin in front of my waist. What a procedure!

I turned and faced myself in the vanity mirror above my washbasin. It was a moment I'll never forget. I thought of Sue's sister Wendy, whose uniform I'd always coveted. I thought of all the nurses I'd been impressed by at the hospital. I pictured them soothing brows, pushing trolleys, calming anxious relatives and offering tea in pale green cups and saucers that matched their dresses. Now, in this moment, I saw myself amongst their ranks. 'I really am becoming an MRI nurse!' I said to my surprised reflection.

When Nessa and Linda arrived a few minutes later we all shrieked and hugged each other.

'Will you look at the state of us!' Linda exclaimed as we 'oohed' and 'aahed' over each other like bridesmaids before a wedding.

Nessa and I both knew she was feeling exactly the same as us, though: pleased as punch and bubbling with pride.

Sharing such exciting new experiences with the other girls helped me through the first few weeks, although I still felt horribly homesick. Graham visited a couple of times a week, turning up in the hospital car park in his bubble car and taking me into Manchester for a cup of coffee and a chat. Once or twice he drove me home to visit my parents at the weekends, too, but I'm not sure that helped my feelings of homesickness as I always found it very hard to say goodbye to them.

Several weeks on, after my eight-week school-based 'block' was complete, I reported for ward duty for the first time with Sister Craddock, who paired me with an efficient-looking third-year student called Maggie. I was assured Maggie would ably instruct me in the arts of completing a bedpan and bottle round and giving bed baths, and I couldn't wait to get started.

'Most patients can manage by themselves if you draw the curtain and give them a bottle or a bedpan,' Maggie said brightly, which immediately put me at my ease. She had already dished out half a dozen stainless steel bedpans, and she asked me to follow her round the ward and help her collect them by placing a paper cover on them and loading them on a trolley.

'Nobody likes this job,' she said as we went into the sluice. 'The golden rule is to look the other way and stand back so you don't splatter your apron.'

There was a porcelain sink on the back wall, into which Maggie tipped the contents of the pans before flushing the metal chain that was dangling beside it. The smell that rose up my nostrils as the urine and faeces were washed away made me heave, and I held my breath.

Maggie turned on the taps on either side of the sink and swilled out the pans before loading them one at a time into a sterilising unit that looked like a narrow metal washing machine. Each bedpan was blasted with boiling, steamy water before Maggie removed it with a thick linen cloth and placed it on a clean trolley ready for the next bedpan round.

'The trick is to get it over and done with as quickly as you can,' Maggie said. 'Grit your teeth and just do it. If there's one thing I've learned it's that bedpans won't clean themselves and, believe me, the smell gets worse the longer you leave it!'

I felt at ease with Maggie and hung on her every word, eager to learn from her experience. Our next task was to perform a bed bath on Mr Finch.

'He's a good one to start with as he lives up to his name and is as light as a bird,' Maggie whispered as we approached his bed.

'Good day, Nurses!' Mr Finch beamed as Maggie pushed a trolley beside his bed and I closed the curtains around him. 'Is it bathtime? Oh, go on then, if y'insist!'

Mr Finch put down his *Daily Mirror* and rubbed his hands together cheekily, eyes glinting.

'He's just teasing,' Maggie said. 'Aren't you, Mr Finch?'

'I am indeed,' he tittered. 'I'm a good boy really.'

Maggie caught my eye and winked, but I still felt slightly nervous. Mr Finch looked a bit scruffy, with nicotine-stained fingers and blackened teeth, and I shivered as I wondered what we might have to deal with under the sheets.

'Any trouble from him, Nurse Lawton, and we'll make sure the water is ice cold next time,' Maggie said in an exaggerated whisper.

On the trolley Maggie had a pot of zinc and castor oil cream, a metal bowl filled with warm water and a tin of talcum powder. Mr Finch reached into his locker and produced a toilet bag containing a bar of Palmolive soap, two grey flannels and a small, thin towel.

Maggie showed me how to strip the counterpane back and pull the blanket off the patient and over an A-shaped frame she had placed at the foot of the bed.

'Keep the top sheet in place and work underneath it as best you can,' Maggie said quietly. 'That's the privacy guard.'

She demonstrated by washing and drying Mr Finch's face first and moving on to his arms, chest and underarms without exposing an inch of flesh unnecessarily.

'Ooh, that's grand, Nurse,' Mr Finch commented. 'You're right good at this!'

Next I helped turn Mr Finch on his side, so Maggie could wash down his back and I could dry it. He certainly was as light as a bird. He was skin and bone, in fact, and I realised he looked rather like the old man in the television comedy *Steptoe and Son*, which amused me.

'Would you wash your private bits?' Maggie said, making it sound as though she was posing a question when in actual fact she was instructing Mr Finch politely to do so.

'Course,' he said. 'I tell ye what, it's a damn sight easier t' get m'self clean nowadays. Used to be murder when I were down the pit.'

It turned out that Mr Finch was born at the turn of the century and had worked nearly all his life at the Astley Green Colliery in Wigan, mining coal for decades until his retirement a few years earlier. He had seven children and seventeen grandchildren, and had served in both world wars.

As Maggie and I rolled him onto each side again so we could strip and re-make the bed beneath him, I thought how silly I was to have been nervous about him, and how unkind I was to have assumed he might be smelly or uncouth, just because he was old and had spent his life working his fingers to the bone.

I loved getting to know such interesting folk and I soon realised that once people are stripped bare in a hospital bed, that's when you find out who they really are. This realisation struck me as so profound that I wrote it down in my notebook when I returned to my room after tea, because I never wanted to forget it. As I did so, I realised with some satisfaction that despite still being plagued by homesickness, and despite feeling mentally and physically drained at the end of the day, I was doing my very best and I was slowly starting to find my feet.

I fell into an extremely deep sleep that night. Sister Mary Francis would have called it the 'sleep of the just', but my much-needed slumber was suddenly interrupted when an alarm bell rang out. In my dream I saw a ghostly-white patient desperately pressing a red emergency buzzer. I couldn't see the patient's face and I didn't know which ward he was on or what was wrong with him. I could see him holding out his hands to me, but I couldn't get close enough to help him because I was stuck behind a pile of textbooks that towered higher and higher the more I tried to move forwards. Physiology. Anatomy. Dietetics. Bacteriology. The words swarmed, distorting my vision.

'Wake up, Linda! Get up quick!' It was Anne's voice, and she was hammering on my door. 'There's a fire! Get up!'

I stumbled out of bed, my heart thumping. The alarm in my dream suddenly got louder and louder. My door was open now and I could see nurses running towards the emergency exit along the corridor. The fire alarm was blasting out as I grabbed my dressing gown and ran, barefoot, into the arms of a burly fireman.

'Steady now!' he grinned. 'There's no need to panic. Just make your way outside calmly and we should be able to get you back inside in no time at all.'

We were told a small fire had broken out on the opposite side of the nurses' home, which was soon contained. This news travelled quickly around the car park, where I stood shivering in my nightie and dressing gown, still feeling drugged by sleep. Eventually another very handsome fireman led me back to my room, which he was in the process of checking over when the home sister stuck her nose round my door.

'See that you remove that poster in the morning,' she said huffily, pointing to my beloved black and white John Lennon portrait taped boldly above my bed. 'You know quite well it is forbidden to decorate the walls.'

The fireman flashed me a dazzling smile and rolled his eyes behind her back before wishing me a very good night.

'Do you know, I think I'll always have a soft spot for firemen,' I told Anne dreamily at breakfast the next morning.

'All the more reason to work hard,' Anne replied with a wink. 'Everyone knows firemen have a soft spot for nurses, too.'

'You're right,' I smiled. 'Perhaps I've chosen the right career after all!'

Chapter Three

*'I didn't expect to be looking after people
who are actually ill'*

'Lawton, attend to Mrs Roache in bed thirteen,' Sister
Bridie ordered. I hated the way she addressed us by our
surnames, as if we were in the Army. I leapt to attention,
nevertheless.

I was now a good few months into my first year of training.
So far I'd had a trouble-free start to my nursing career. Soon
after the eight weeks of study with Mr Tate, which were punctuated by visits to wards and units, I completed my first placement, which happened to be at the eye hospital over the road
in Nelson Street.

We had no say in where we were sent for work experience,
but I had no complaints and was quite happy dishing out eye
drops, wiping down lockers and fetching cups of tea for
patients, while at the same time learning how to sterilise
equipment, organise the linen cupboard and generally keep
Sister happy.

The only part of the work that worried me at the eye hospital was using the sterilising equipment. The machine was
different to the bedpan steriliser I'd become accustomed to
operating in the sluices at the main hospital. This one stood on
a substantial trolley that was positioned right in the middle of
the ward. It looked harmless enough, shaped like a small

stainless-steel oven, but it hissed and bubbled as loudly as a witch's cauldron.

I'd seen other nurses adeptly sterilising kidney bowls, syringes and needles, seemingly oblivious to the dangers of the swirling clouds of hot steam the contraption emitted whenever it was opened, but I was scared to death the first time I had to operate it by myself, jumping back in fright as the sweltering steam billowed into my face. I practically threw the instruments in, pulling my hand away and slamming the door shut in record time. It was a miracle I hadn't been burned, especially as I had to repeat the process in reverse five minutes later, retrieving my poker-hot equipment with a pair of Cheatle forceps.

Needless to say, I soon got used to the steriliser, and by the time I left the eye unit I think I could have operated it in my sleep. My next placement was to be on Sister Bridie's surgical ward.

'Are you looking forward to it?' Graham asked me the night before I was to start there, when he picked me up in his car and took me out for a coffee at a little snack bar in Piccadilly Gardens, up near the station.

'Oh yes,' I replied. 'Very much so. The eye unit was good experience but it wasn't exactly exciting.' The fierce steriliser had been the only thing that made my pulse quicken. 'I'm ready for the next challenge. A surgical ward should be very interesting. It's a female ward and I expect women need surgery for all sorts of reasons. It'll be good to deal with more than just eyes.'

'That's my little nurse!' Graham said encouragingly.

'I'm a bit worried about Sister Bridie, though,' I admitted. 'She's Irish and a spinster, so I hear, and she seems terribly strict and bossy.'

'Don't fret. You were worried about the Matron to begin with,' Graham reminded me, 'and I've hardly heard you mention her since.'

'That's true,' I said thoughtfully. 'I guess I've learned that Miss Morgan leaves you alone as long as you keep your head, and your skirt length, down!'

'Glad to hear it,' he smiled.

'Besides, you always know when Matron is on the warpath, as word spreads like Chinese whispers. "Matron's coming, pass it on," we say, and usually the entire ward is on best behaviour before she has set foot through the main doors.'

Sister Bridie worried me more, I realised. 'I'll be seeing her on a daily basis on the surgical ward, come what may. I've heard she used to be on the men's cardiac ward, and she shouted so loudly at the student nurses that she nearly gave the patients another heart attack.'

Graham laughed and I joined in, seeing through his eyes how funny this was. He was a marvellous help to me. Despite the camaraderie I shared with Linda and the other girls and the endless encouragement offered by my mum on the phone and on my occasional weekend visits home, it was Graham who kept me going, always willing to drive up to the hospital two or even three times a week to see me and let me unload about my day.

Sometimes I cried in his arms as we huddled together in the hospital car park, because I was tired out and I missed him and my home so much. Graham always provided a good reason for me to keep my chin up and carry on. 'Think how you'll feel when you're a qualified SRN,' he would say. 'We'll be able to get married and get a place of our own! You've come this far. You can do it, Linda. I'm so proud of you. You were made for this job.'

Now he commented: 'I can't imagine you giving Sister Bridie any reason whatsoever to shout at you.'

I hoped he was right, and his words helped set my mind at ease a little. All I had to do was obey orders and work hard, and I had nothing to fear. 'What doesn't kill me will make me stronger,' I thought.

Graham also used to chat to me about events in the news and life outside the hospital, which helped to put things in perspective. I was so wrapped up in my own life I hardly ever took time to read a newspaper. Sometimes I didn't even breathe fresh air for days on end, as the nurses' home was attached to the main hospital by a covered walkway. Graham was my reality check, my link to the outside world.

'Life is full of ups and downs, Linda,' he said. 'You have to take the rough with the smooth. Look at it like this. One minute the country is on a huge high, ruling the world with the football. The next, something terrible happens, like the Aberfan disaster. That's life.'

It was just a few months since England had won the World Cup in the summer of 1966. I'm not a football fan, but I remembered Graham proudly telling me that Geoff Hurst, our hat-trick-scoring striker, was a local man who had been born in Ashton. Then in October the terrible Aberfan tragedy had united the country in the most dreadful grief. More than 100 children perished in that Welsh village when a slag heap collapsed on their school.

Life can be very cruel, and plenty of people had it a lot harder than me; that was an absolute certainty. In the big scheme of things, Sister Bridie's harsh tongue was scarcely a hardship, and I resolved to do my very best under her watchful eye.

The night before my placement on the surgical ward began I noted in my diary that, thanks to my gentle introduction to basic nursing at the eye unit, as well as Graham's words of wisdom and encouragement, I was feeling much more settled, and my confidence was slowly building.

> The hospital and nurses' home are now very familiar, and the strict regimes bring a sense of order and security, which I find comforting. Graham hasn't actually ever proposed to me properly, but I like it when he suggests we'll get married one day, and settle down. I would like that very much. I have learned that I prize security over uncertainty, and I want to pass my exams and qualify, because then my future will be set.

'Lawton, attend to Mrs Roache in bed thirteen,' Sister Bridie repeated impatiently, even though I was already picking up the notes to obey the order.

'Yes, Sister,' I said politely, giving her a nod. 'Right away, Sister.'

I thought about being strong and making Graham proud as I strode to the far end of the surgical ward. I didn't want to make any mistakes here. Sister Bridie had split purple veins etched across her grey complexion. Her silver hair was wrapped in a tight bun and a single white whisker protruded from a stone-like mole on her chin. She was as round and squat as a concrete mixer, and when she barked orders it felt as if she was spitting gravel at me. Sister Bridie was not a person I wanted to cross.

I hadn't been prepared for the strong smell on the surgical ward, like nothing I'd ever encountered before. It clung in the air, and I found myself trying to take short, shallow breaths through my nose so as not to experience the full stench. Breathing like that made me tense my neck, and I could feel my starched white collar tighten around my throat, making me slightly light-headed. I remembered Janice telling us how she had embarrassed herself by gagging violently in front of the patients when she had to collect used bedpans on her first placement, but this smell was different and at first I couldn't identify it.

I could hear trolleys rattling hurriedly past, Sister Bridie pebbling other nurses with orders and the unmistakable, upsetting sound of ladies crying out in pain. Against this background noise, all I could think about was the inescapable smell sticking to every pore on my skin. It made me clench my insides, to try and stop the smell getting through to me.

Mrs Roache was lying on her back with her right leg in traction. She had been hit by a speeding car as she crossed the Stretford Road in Hulme to collect her pension, and her thigh bone was very badly smashed. The old lady was on powerful drugs to help her cope with the considerable pain. Her leg had been dressed and strapped into what I recognised as a Thomas splint, which ran from beneath her pelvis right down to her ankle. Poor soul, I thought. She looked a sorry sight, propped up on top of her bedclothes, her blue-rinsed hair still matted into an ugly gash in her scalp.

'How are you, Mrs Roache?' I smiled as I approached her bedside. She was a generously proportioned lady who gamely attempted a smile, but her pain got the better of her. 'Been better, t' be honest, Nurse,' she struggled. 'Can I have some more p-p-painkillers?' She winced as she squeezed her lips together to suppress a moan.

'That's why I'm here,' I soothed. 'You're ready for your next dose. If you'll just allow me to help you tilt your head, I'll pass you a fresh glass of water.'

I offered words of encouragement as she eagerly placed the two pellet-like pills in her mouth and swallowed them down in one tremendous gulp. I had learned that it is not uncommon for patients to be sick after taking painkilling drugs, and I had brought a vomit bowl with me, which I was holding in my hand.

'They should start to work quite quickly ...' I began, but I was promptly silenced by the sight of Mrs Roache simultaneously retching and lurching towards me.

I froze and looked on in helpless horror as she valiantly aimed for the metal bowl but missed it completely. Instead, she vomited right the way down my arm, splattering the sleeve of my uniform, my cuff and my bare forearm simultaneously. The sight and smell of her vomit, not to mention the warm feel of it clinging to my skin, made my own insides churn. As Mrs Roache was sick again, this time directly into the metal bowl I'd let drop beside her, I threw up the contents of my own stomach right into the same receptacle.

'I'm ever so sorry, Nurse ...' Mrs Roache apologised. She looked ashamed and forlorn, and I didn't want her to suffer any further distress.

'It's no bother. I'm sorry too.' I wiped my face with the hem of my apron and took a slow, deep breath to gather my composure before I began to mop up Mrs Roache's chin with a tissue from her locker. 'What a pair we are,' I smiled at her. Nausea was swimming through my insides now and I desperately hoped I wouldn't be sick again. 'Give me a minute to clean myself up and we'll start again, shall we?'

'Thank you, Nurse, I'm ever so sorry,' she said as I walked unsteadily to the sluice to dispose of the contents of the sick bowl.

I was burning with a mixture of emotions. I felt sorry for the poor old lady, who had suffered the most appalling injury, and I felt mortified by what had happened. My cheeks flushed and I found myself saying a little prayer in my head, and imagining God was holding my hand. This was something Sister Mary Francis had encouraged us to do at school whenever we needed a little help and guidance.

'Dear God,' I began as I held my nose and emptied the vomit into the sluice. 'Please help me to be strong. This job is going to be harder than I imagined.'

I heaved, changed my apron and headed back to attend to Mrs Roache again. Sister Bridie was patrolling the ward now, and I had to look competent and in control, though I felt anything but.

In the bed next to Mrs Roache lay a distinguished-looking elderly lady called Mrs Pearlman. If my memory served me correctly, the patient notes I'd seen when I arrived on the ward told me she was Jewish, and she had a fractured pelvis.

She raised a thin arm to attract my attention. I stepped towards her with a smile and said, 'How can I help? I'll be with you just as soon as I've finished with Mrs Roache ...'

'There is no need, my dear,' she said in a raspy whisper. 'I just wanted to say I think you are doing a *marvellous* job.'

I felt humbled.

That night I sat on my bed and cried. I'd had a long soak in the bath but I was sure I could still smell poor Mrs Roache's vomit on my skin. It mingled with the scent of the powdered Ajax and Lysol cleaning liquid we used on the wards, and the medicated pong of Izal toilet paper that hung in the air around all the communal bathrooms and toilets in the nurses' home.

I was scrubbing my hair with Sunsilk shampoo for the third time when there was a knock on the bathroom door from Anne, who was politely wondering if she could possibly hurry me up so she could 'de-hospitalise' herself as well.

Her words made me think of the putrid smell that hung in the air on the surgical ward and I suddenly realised why it was worse than the usual hospital smell I was used to: it was gangrene. I hadn't been able to identify it because I'd never smelled anything like it in my life before, but now it all became horribly clear. Mr Tate had explained that antibiotics were used to help prevent gangrene setting in, but they did not always manage the job. I remembered his words clearly and recalled wincing when he told us: 'Gangrene occurs when body tissue and cells are no longer receiving blood flow and oxygen, and those parts of the body effectively die and emit a fetid smell.'

I was not familiar with the word 'fetid', though it was obvious it meant something unpleasant. As he spoke, Mr Tate was squeezing his upper lip between his thumb and forefinger, as he had a habit of doing, and I remembered feeling slightly queasy.

Now I felt a wave of sickness crash in my stomach all over again. I was so clean my skin was pink and shining, yet I still felt infected with bad odours. Fetid, I realised, was a polite way of describing the stench of rotting flesh. The patients on that ward had suffered horrific injuries. Beneath the assorted splints and dressings and Plasters of Paris, parts of their bodies were dying. I was repulsed. This job really was much harder than I'd thought it was going to be.

I cried and cried for hours that night, longing to go home so much it physically hurt. I had a deep pain in my chest. Each rib had hardened around my lungs and each breath I drew made me ache more.

Perhaps I could pack my suitcase and slip quietly out of the hospital in the morning? I allowed myself that fantasy, watching myself, in my mind's eye, grappling with the heavy drawers of my wardrobe, removing my clothes silently and running off. I would leave my uniform behind, and as I slipped away Miss Morgan and Sister Bridie would become small, insignificant grey dots in the distance, never to be seen again. 'I'm going home to my mum!' I would shout, waving my John Lennon poster brazenly in my hand.

I knew it couldn't happen like that. Even though I was still a very young eighteen-year-old, I was wise enough to realise there would have to be meetings and confrontations, soul-searching and contingency plans.

What would I do instead of nursing? How could I let everyone down? My parents were so pleased I had entered not only a respected profession, but the magnificent institution that was the NHS. They were delighted I would earn such luxuries as a staff pension and holiday pay, benefits not available to them as they were self-employed. I couldn't upset them, certainly not without a back-up plan. Perhaps I should look into nursery nursing, which had crossed my mind when I first considered nursing. I imagined working with children would be a much more enjoyable job, but how could I change course now?

Graham would be so disappointed if I gave up nursing. He had joined the police force from school and had wanted to rise through the ranks, but health problems prevented him from fulfilling his ambition. Now he was making a very good job of selling second-hand cars, like his father, and he wanted the world for me. He would be sad if his little nurse faltered and failed, despite his optimistic predictions.

As I tucked myself in and lay awake in the dark, I felt another emotion: shame. I felt ashamed of myself for wanting to quit. I thought of poor Mrs Roache, paralysed in her hospital bed, unable to take control of her own destiny. She had been knocked down by a car and was in agony, but still she tried to smile at me. Still she made an effort. That's what I had to do.

'Please promise me, Linda, that you will always work hard for your living.' I heard Sister Mary Francis's words as I nodded off to sleep, and I told myself to keep going, just keep going.

The following week Nessa, Anne, Jo, Linda, Janice and I assembled in the schoolroom for some practical work. We were to be shown how to use a Ryles tube, which caused great excitement as we all enjoyed having hands-on experience. It meant we were progressing, taking another step closer to becoming qualified nurses, without the daunting pressure of being on the wards.

'How are you getting on?' Jo asked while we waited for Mr Tate to fetch the tubes from the store cupboard. We'd been so busy working on our separate placements, as well as studying, that it had been weeks since we'd had a proper catch-up. In the evenings we were completely exhausted, and all we wanted to do was get to bed as soon as possible to make the early starts more bearable.

'I'm all right,' I said, giving a thin, unconvincing smile. 'The surgical ward with Sister Bridie is tough, though. I didn't expect to be looking after people who are actually ill.'

I hadn't meant to make a joke but Jo sniggered. 'What *did* you expect?' she asked, then added, 'I know what you mean. I had no idea what I was letting myself in for either, not really. At the start I couldn't see why we needed ten aprons, but I certainly do now. I've had two of mine covered in unmentionable bodily waste already this week. It's disgusting!'

Jo explained that she'd done a bedpan round on the cardiac ward and had misjudged how full one of the covered metal pans was when she carried it rather too hastily to the sluice.

'I think the poor man must have been hanging on to that lot for a week,' she said, holding her nose dramatically and pretending to gag.

'Once I'd changed and collected the next set of pans from the other side of the ward, I then managed to splatter myself in hot, orange-coloured urine. It was toxic, I swear!'

'Yuk!' I said, thinking Mrs Roache's vomit didn't seem quite so repulsive after all. 'At least you can laugh about it.'

'Needs must,' Jo replied, somewhat begrudgingly.

Linda was looking very pleased with herself and couldn't wait to tell us she had given her first injection the day before, which we were all quite jealous of.

'What was it like?' we chirped.

'It was as easy as pie,' she beamed. 'Mind you, thanks to Sister Barnes I did have a whale of a man as my first victim. He said he didn't feel a thing, which was hardly surprising with all that blubber on his backside!'

Sister Barnes was my favourite sister. I'd spent several days between placements helping out on her orthopaedic ward, and every time I saw her she was smiling. She was big and blonde and, unlike practically all the other sisters, she had a man-friend whom she mentioned often and was clearly very much in love with. Her happiness seemed to rub off on those around her and she had a wonderful, calming influence on her staff and patients alike.

I learned from a third year that Sister Barnes had trained at the MRI and was still in her thirties, making her one of the youngest sisters I encountered. She always made herself available to us young students, telling us that she remembered her own training well and was there to help. If we had any questions whatsoever, we were to knock on her door and simply ask.

I admired Sister Barnes and, despite my difficulties, I aspired to be like her. How wonderful it would be to become a successful sister like her, and inspire students in the way she inspired me! The thought cheered me up. Hospital life was tough, but that didn't mean I couldn't make a success of it and come out smiling, just like Sister Barnes.

I listened attentively as Mr Tate dished out the narrow plastic Ryles tubes, which he explained were used either to deliver liquid food to the patient, or to 'aspirate' or empty the stomach contents, typically before an operation.

'I want you to practise in pairs,' he said. 'Nurse Lawton and Nurse Maudsley, here are your tubes.'

Jo and I looked at each other cautiously, but were secretly quite thrilled about this lesson. If we were to be let loose on the patients with Ryles tubes, we knew we must have earned some trust and respect from our superiors, and were progressing well.

'Please watch very carefully,' Mr Tate continued. He picked out a student from another group, a fashionable-looking girl called Cynthia Weaver, and he set about demonstrating how to insert the thin tube into her nose and throat and then gently down into her stomach.

As she lay with her head on a pillow on a low couch, I could see Cynthia clench her fists and bite her lips until they went blue as Mr Tate threaded and teased the tube patiently up her right nostril. He gave a running commentary about the amount of force and manipulation required at each stage.

There was no need for him to tell us when it had reached Cynthia's throat and stomach because she gagged and wriggled uncomfortably, her silky bobbed hair dancing around the pillow.

It was my turn to be a 'patient' next, and I was thankful to have Jo, whose self-confidence never faltered, as my 'nurse'. She proved quite adept at navigating my nasal passage and manoeuvring the tube down my throat, and I was surprised to find it didn't hurt one bit. The sensation was completely alien to me, though, and my eyes watered and I began to heave as it passed down into my stomach.

'Mission accomplished,' Jo said triumphantly, while I swallowed a whole pint of water in record time to lessen the sensation and keep the tube in place long enough for Mr Tate to acknowledge Jo's work.

I found it surprisingly easy to replicate the process the other way round, and Mr Tate congratulated us on our efforts. 'Well done,' he said. 'Textbook work.' He was always succinct in his praise, but it meant a great deal.

Janice and Nessa were paired together, and I noticed they were both very quiet. This wasn't unusual for Nessa. She was probably the cleverest of us all and was always diligently focused on the job in hand. Janice, however, didn't look her normal assured self.

'Are you OK?' I asked as we sat down later in the canteen.

We each had a plate of unidentifiable meat, grey mashed potato and pellet-like peas. It looked totally unappetising, but we usually managed to eat a huge helping of food at each sitting, followed by a steaming pudding with lumpy custard you could stand your spoon up in. No matter what it looked like we tucked in, knowing we needed all the energy we could get through the day.

'Fine, I suppose,' Janice replied as she forked her food into her mouth robotically and stared into space. There was a moment of silence before she added, 'To tell the truth, I'm not sure this is the career for me.' Pushing her half-eaten meal away she shrugged her shoulders and asked, 'How about you?'

'A bit the same, I suppose,' I found myself reluctantly admitting. 'When I did my first placement at the eye unit, I thought I was fine. The worst thing I ever saw was someone's eyeball dangling on their cheek. The rest of it was all putting on eye patches, administering eye drops, sterilising needles, taking people to the toilet, helping them into the bath. They weren't ill, not physically ill. Now it's all gangrene and vomit and pain and suffering, I'm finding it hard.'

Janice surveyed me. 'I think we're different,' she said. 'You're a naturally caring person, Linda. You've got what it takes. I can't even stomach helping people have a bath or go to the loo. How can you touch their bodies and wipe their behinds? I just can't do it.'

I had never seen a man naked until I worked in the eye unit. Even Graham's body remained something of a mystery to me, though we'd been together for well over a year by now. A bit of hanky-panky was allowed but nice girls waited until they were married before having sex; that's how I was brought up. Despite living such a sheltered life, naked bodies didn't alarm me in the slightest, and it had never occurred to me to be squeamish about bodily functions. I had taken it in my stride and focused on what I could do to help the patients, not how I felt to see them with no clothes on.

Perhaps Janice was right, I considered. Perhaps I did have what it took to be a real nurse, but I think I still needed some convincing.

Back on the surgical ward the following week, I was relieved to be given the mundane task of tidying and wiping down lockers, disposing of wilting flowers and filling up water jugs. This gave me the chance to chat to some of the patients.

Mercifully, Mrs Roache was lying in what appeared to be a comfortable slumber, though how she managed it with that enormous splint on her leg I never knew. Mrs Pearlman, however, was wide awake in the next bed.

'How are you, my dear?' she asked me kindly. 'You girls do work so very hard. We're lucky to have such angels as you to care for us.'

Mrs Pearlman was a wonderful old lady. Well into her seventies, she lived alone after being widowed many years earlier, and had fallen down the stairs of her old miner's cottage in Hazel Grove. Her pelvis was fractured in several places and she had been in hospital for weeks on end. She never had many visitors and I was amazed at how she remained so positive.

'I'm very well, Mrs Pearlman,' I replied. 'How are you today?'

'Fine, dear, just fine. I think the care I'm receiving here is absolutely first class. Do you know what is on the menu today? I had the most delicious roast chicken yesterday, and a roll of ice cream that melted in my mouth. Isn't the NHS the most marvellous institution?'

Mrs Pearlman did wonders for my spirits, and I made a point of chatting to her every day. She wore a beautifully embroidered bed jacket and often asked me to comb her surprisingly thick hair, which was dyed jet black but now had silver roots showing.

In her day, I imagined she had been an immaculately groomed, fine figure of a lady, the sort who might run the local Women's Institute group or sing in the choral society. I marvelled at how graciously she accepted her fate, lying in this bed, silver roots creeping longer by the day.

'Lawton, there are three beds to be made. Help Bennyon.'

The Irish voice was sharp and it made my nerves snap. 'Yes, Sister Bridie,' I said, nodding a polite goodbye to Mrs Pearlman and scuttling to the other end of the ward, where Lesley Bennyon, a friendly second-year student, was holding a pile of linen.

'Three gone in the night,' she said sadly, eyeing the empty beds. 'Mrs Hall, Mrs Atherton and Mrs Lloyd.'

Their faces flashed before me. All were frail and elderly and had a collection of badly broken wrists, ribs and collar-bones between them. I opened my mouth to speak but no words came out. I wanted to say 'I hope they didn't suffer,' but I knew, from the infections and smells and disturbing noises that inhabited this corner of the ward, that was highly unlikely.

'It was their time,' Lesley said softly, filling the silence.

Together we made the fresh beds with impressive speed, checking the corners of the sheets were tightly tucked and the counterpanes perfectly parallel, turning the pillowcase ends away from the ward door and twisting the wheels so they faced into the bed, for neatness and safety.

'Neatness and safety,' Lesley hissed to me, mimicking Sister Bridie's Irish lilt. 'You have to be neat and you have to be safe, to be sure! Don't ever forget that, Lawton, or you'll be struck down dead like these poor unfortunate ladies here, God rest their souls.'

I could sense Lesley had a soft heart and that this was simply her way of dealing with death.

'You have to laugh,' she said. 'Or you'd spend the whole time crying.'

Despite being upset I gave a little laugh too, letting some of my tension escape, as Lesley wanted me to. Just then she leapt up unexpectedly and gave a little scream.

'Arrgh! Not again!' She rubbed her hands up and down her thighs and laughed awkwardly, as you do when you knock your funny bone. I leaned across the bed to place my arm on hers, to ask if she was OK, and suddenly I sprang up too, shooting inches into the air. A mild electric shock had run all the way through my body and, like Lesley, I instinctively began to rub my thighs, half-laughing and half-moaning.

'It's these ruddy suspender belts,' Lesley winced. 'Iron beds, prickly blankets and metal clasps on suspender belts are a lethal combination. Making beds in stockings should carry a "high voltage" warning! Come on, let's go and sort out the linen cupboard. I think we've earned it.'

She gave me a little wink and I followed her through the ward and into the large linen store near the main doors. This was a godsend, I'd learned. Each ward had one, and it was a little haven where you could make yourself look busy and hide from Sister whenever you needed a breather.

'Have you heard the gossip?' Lesley asked when we were safely inside. She handed me a stack of pillowcases to fold, though they were already in a fairly neat pile. I was all ears.

'Cassie Webster and Sharon Carter have been suspended for a month for stealing bread from the dining room.'

'Never!' I exclaimed, genuinely shocked. The hospital food was truly terrible. We lived on a diet of rubbery eggs and greasy strips of bacon for breakfast and the ubiquitous lumpy mash and unidentifiable meat for lunch and dinner. Afternoon tea was the only enjoyable offering of the day, when we had tea and fairy cakes and freshly baked Hovis loaves, which we slathered with jam and butter. Everyone tried to get to the first sitting for afternoon tea, else there wouldn't be much left, but I'd never heard of anyone stealing the bread before.

'Seems they fancied taking a couple of Hovis loaves back to their flat with them, and Matron, of all people, caught them red-handed! Walked right into them, apparently, as they smuggled them out the door, still warm and wrapped in their aprons!'

I gulped as Lesley continued the tale, knowing how seriously this offence would be viewed. 'Matron was purple with rage as she marched them to her office, shouting as she did so. Nancy Porter heard every word and it's gone all over the hospital!'

Lesley jutted out her chin, pursed her lips and pushed out her chest, Miss Morgan-style. 'You have stained your reputations as upstanding, trustworthy young ladies!' she mimicked. 'Your mothers will be distraught when they find out about this disgraceful carry-on. Do not darken the door of the MRI for one month. You are suspended with immediate effect. Take the time to contemplate the error of your ways.'

'Shhhhh!' hissed a young nurse I'd never seen before, who suddenly loomed in the linen cupboard doorway. 'I can hear you on the ward – and Matron's coming!'

Lesley and I both fell into a heap, stuffing flannels between our teeth to stifle our laughter. We hid behind the door until the sound of Matron's clicking heels subsided. We'd had a lucky escape and we wanted to keep it that way, so we held our breath as we strained to hear her distant tones telling some poor soul to report to her office at once. 'It appears you need a reminder ...' we heard Matron saying before her voice faded away. No doubt she was going to deliver a lecture about skirt lengths or tidy hair, her two bugbears.

Before I finished my shift that day I went to see Mrs Pearlman.

'Hello, my dear, I'm glad you've come,' she said. 'I have something for you.' She reached for an elegant gold watch that was lying on top of her locker and held it out to me.

'Oh, I couldn't possibly ...' I began. I had never seen the watch before and I knew patients were not meant to have valuables lying about the place. I was pretty sure nurses were not meant to accept gifts like this from patients, either. I'd seen Sister Gorton confiscating bottles of sherry given as gifts to nurses at the eye unit, though rumour did have it that she was 'fond of her drink' and took the bottles home with her, whereupon they were never seen again.

'Please take it,' Mrs Pearlman said, clutching my hand and curling the watch into my palm. 'You will make an elderly lady very happy. I want you to have it.'

I smiled and nodded awkwardly, slipping it into my pocket before thanking Mrs Pearlman politely and wishing her a good night. As I walked out of the ward I felt very uncomfortable. I imagined Matron striding up to me, her X-ray eyes zooming in on the gold in my pocket. 'Explain yourself!' she would bellow, I was sure of it. What if she thought I'd stolen the watch from Mrs Pearlman? My blood ran cold, and I decided to drop by Sister Barnes's office on my way out, to ask her advice.

When I laid the watch on the table before Sister Barnes, I felt instant relief. 'I didn't want to offend her, but now I don't know what to do,' I explained.

'You've done exactly the right thing in coming to see me,' Sister Barnes smiled. 'A small box of chocolates at Christmas is one thing, but a gift like this is something else. Your instincts are quite correct. I'm afraid you will have to return the watch to Mrs Pearlman and explain that, although you are very touched by her generous gesture, it is against the rules to accept gifts from patients, and you are sure she will understand that you do not wish to get into trouble.'

I exhaled rather more loudly than I meant to, releasing my stress.

'How are you getting on?' Sister Barnes asked thoughtfully.

'Fine,' I said.

'Just fine?' She raised an eyebrow quizzically.

'Yes, it's just … it's harder than I thought it would be.'

'I remember thinking the very same thing when I was your age,' she replied. 'You need to believe in yourself more. I think you have what it takes, but do you?'

I felt very small and meek besides Sister Barnes. My shoulders were hunched, my chin was lowered and I felt washed out with tiredness. She, on the other hand, looked vibrant and full of life. Her eyes were twinkling, and she had an energy about her that made me want to straighten my spine and pull my shoulders back.

Sister Barnes eyed me thoughtfully and then stood up and clapped her hands together twice, as if struck by a bright idea.

'Come with me,' she said cheerfully. 'Wash your hands and put your apron back on. I have a patient who needs an injection, and I think you are exactly the right nurse for the job.'

My heart leapt. I'd been desperate to give someone an injection ever since I arrived, but until now the opportunity hadn't presented itself. Sister Barnes was young enough to remember how much it means to a young student nurse to be trusted with a syringe and a vial of drugs for the first time. I was thrilled.

As soon as I saw the patient in question I allowed myself a wry smile, remembering Linda's description of the whale-like patient who was her first 'victim'. Mrs Butcher was the female equivalent and I knew exactly why clever Sister Barnes had decided to let me loose on this particular patient.

'Mrs Butcher, Nurse Lawton is here to give you your injection,' Sister Barnes announced as she pulled the curtain around the bed and asked Mrs Butcher to lift her nightdress and present her right buttock.

'Is it the first time she's given an injection?' Mrs Butcher asked, surveying me suspiciously, no doubt because I looked so young.

'Not at all,' Sister Barnes replied. 'This is a demonstration to show how proficient Nurse Lawton is.'

Mrs Butcher sniffed and rolled over clumsily while I reminded myself to seek out the upper, outer quadrant of the buttock as I'd been taught during our practice on oranges in the classroom. Moments later, I pushed the needle through

Mrs Butcher's extremely well-padded rump and administered the drug steadily, with surprising ease.

'All done!' I said triumphantly. I tingled inside. I felt absolutely fantastic.

'Didn't feel a thing!' beamed Mrs Butcher, her face cracking into a satisfied smile.

'Thank you, Nurse Lawton,' Sister Barnes said. 'Now you can pop back in on Mrs Pearlman before you finish for the day.'

I wanted to skip down the corridor, I felt so exhilarated. I didn't, of course. I walked on the left-hand side, as always, but there was a different rhythm in my step. It felt as though I was bouncing along on fluffy carpets instead of stepping purposefully on the hard stone floor, and I was pretty sure my eyes were twinkling just like Sister Barnes's.

By now, we student nurses had been working flat out for about ten months. Nights out were rare, as we were usually either working, studying or sleeping, but that weekend Linda and I went to a dance at the university. We wore red and yellow mini skirts that Cynthia Weaver had helped us make, after we each bought a strip of fabric in Debenhams. We'd discovered that Cynthia was a very talented dressmaker, making every stitch of her clothing by hand, which is how she managed to always be in the latest fashions. On her advice we teamed the skirts with floral blouses, and I wore my hair in two long plaits, secured with velvet ribbons. As a final touch I doused myself in a generous splash of my favourite perfume, Estée Lauder's *Youth Dew*, cramming the turquoise bottle into my tiny macramé handbag so I could refresh it later.

Strictly speaking, you had to be a university student to go to the dances, but we never had any trouble getting in. Some of the young male students wolf-whistled or messed about making saucy remarks about needing bed baths when we told them we were nurses from the MRI, but it was just light-hearted banter. The students were always happy to help get us in, and would leave us to our own devices once we were through the door.

Sipping orange squash between dances, Linda and I sang along to our favourite records, 'I'm Into Something Good' by Herman's Hermits and 'Bus Stop' by The Hollies. During the evening we gently unloaded on one another too, swapping tales of forgotten bedpans, muddled-up meals and grumpy consultants who mostly seemed to be cast from the same mould and thought the rest of us should treat them like gods.

In contrast, the university students looked as though they didn't have a care in the world. It was as if they had never left school, yet here were Linda and I, on a night out and letting our hair down, yet not quite able to forget about work: the business of life and death.

'So you haven't managed to kill anyone yet?' Linda asked me jokingly, at which I flinched.

'Not quite,' I stuttered.

A month or so earlier I'd had a dreadful experience when I was thrown in at the deep end on one of my first night shifts. I'd pushed it out of my head, but Linda jogged it right back to the forefront of my mind.

'You have to tell me now,' she laughed. 'It's written all over your face!'

'It was awful,' I said. 'I can't believe what happened. I've tried to blot it out!'

'Go on!' she said. 'Get it off your chest.'

'OK,' I said reluctantly. 'Here goes. I was looking after a man called Stanley James, and Sister Craddock had given me strict orders to keep an eye on his fluid intake. He was only allowed an ounce of water hourly, as he was due an operation the next day, and you know what a stickler she is for the intake and output charts.'

Linda rolled her eyes and nodded.

'He begged me for more water but I told him he had to do as Sister ordered, and eventually he settled down to sleep.

'I didn't hear him stir for a while, but when I went to check on him in the early hours I found his flowers on the floor and the empty flower vase in his hands. He looked at me apologetically and said, "I just needed a drink, Nurse."'

Linda gasped. 'He'd drunk the flower water? Oh my God! What happened to him? Did sister blow her stack?'

'She did. I was as terrified of what she would say as I was of what would happen to Mr James. Anyhow, I managed to aspirate most of it back up, but I had to confess all in my report. When Sister Craddock read it, she yelled at me: "He's a very poorly man and you're supposed to be keeping an eye on him." She was so angry her face went red and it made her freckles join up into one big freckle. She kept shouting, "You obviously weren't keeping an eye on him properly!" I thought she was going to suspend me.'

'What happened to Mr James?' Linda asked, eyes bulging.

'He died the next day, unfortunately,' I said. 'Apparently he was a dreadfully ill man and it was unlikely he would have survived for very long, even after the op. That's what Sister Craddock said once she'd calmed down. She was surprisingly understanding, in fact. The flower water wasn't what killed him and she wanted to make that very clear. So to answer your question, Linda, some of my training has been a baptism of fire, but I haven't killed anyone yet! And I'm very glad that Mr James got his last drink before he died.'

We linked arms and walked home at 10.45 p.m. on the dot, to be sure to get in before the 11 p.m. curfew, as the Student Union where the dances were held was on the far side of the vast university campus, about half a mile from the nurses' home. The roads were quiet as usual, save for the occasional Triumph Herald and Hillman Imp that drove by. One cocky young motorist with a head glistening with Brylcreem gave us an admiring wolf-whistle and the offer of a lift, but we politely declined. We broke into fits of giggles as we watched him pull away, leaning over the passenger seat to wind up the window manually, which was impossible to do with any style.

A few students walked in front of us, merrily swaying and singing the song 'We're All Going on a Summer Holiday'. I'd seen the film with Sue at the Stalybridge Palace when it first came out in 1963, and I'd been a big Cliff Richard fan ever since. Graham had even taken me to London to see him in concert with The Shadows at the London Palladium. Watching the students, carefree and clad in brightly coloured drainpipe trousers and winkle-picker shoes, took me right back in time.

'Look at them, they think they're on Carnaby Street!' I joked to Linda, nodding towards the students. She asked about my one and only visit to the capital and I enjoyed reminiscing about it.

I told her Graham and I had gone on a North Western coach from Stalybridge and stayed in a twin room at a rather seedy hotel near the Palladium, though of course we never 'did' anything in the bedroom. Instead, we dutifully went to see the guards at Buckingham Palace and walked hand in hand along Downing Street to pose for a photograph with the policeman outside Number Ten, which every tourist did back then before security was tightened up and the road was sealed off.

After that we strolled along Carnaby Street, admiring the fancy window displays and ultra-fashionable shoppers. London girls wore similar clothes to us – mini skirts, babydoll dresses with matching coloured tights, kinky boots and 'Twiggy' shoes with fancy buckles – but everything seemed exaggerated, somehow. The colours were brighter, the skirts shorter, the belts wider and the shoes shinier – or at least that's how I remembered it. My eyes were on stalks the whole time, and Graham's eyes nearly popped out of his head when he saw the prices of the clothes at the men's outfitters Lord John, as they were far more expensive than in Manchester.

The concert was really great. A kindly usher noticed that Graham and I didn't have a very good view from up in the gods and offered to move us nearer the front. Our new seats were practically on the stage, and when Cliff began to sing I felt as if he was singing just for me. It was very hot and quite stuffy, with dry ice and cigarette smoke filling the air, and by the end of the evening my mustard and black smock dress was thick with perspiration, not to mention the pungent smell of Capstan and Park Drive cigarettes. Graham was so hot he had to remove his tweed jacket and skinny-striped tanktop, but Cliff somehow remained cool and impeccably presented in his sharp-cut suit throughout the show. I adored him!

'We're All Going on a Summer Holiday,' the students on Oxford Road continued to sing badly, jolting me sharply back to this Manchester night in the summer of 1967. I envied the students' freedom, their *joie de vivre*. Just a year or so earlier I had left the Palladium singing that song without a care in the world, just like them. Now life had become much more serious, even though I was still only nineteen years old.

'I guess we all have to grow up some time,' I remarked to Linda wistfully, 'but I feel so old compared to those students!'

'Hey, we're still "Young Ones",' she joshed, recalling another Cliff song, but I think she knew exactly what I meant. We were young, of course, but as student nurses we were no longer carefree.

Chapter Four

'People are dying ... This is harder
than I thought'

One morning about twenty student nurses in my intake assembled in the hospital car park and clambered onto a coach with Mr Tate. Our destination was Booth Hall Children's Hospital in Blackley, north Manchester.

I knew it had a reputation for being one of the finest children's hospitals in the country, and I hung on Mr Tate's every word during the journey as he explained how Humphrey Booth first opened the infirmary in 1908, caring for the sick and destitute from the workhouse after the devastation caused by the plague. In 1914 it took in wounded soldiers from the First World War, and when war was declared a second time the hospital relocated its existing patients and installed a decontamination unit to treat victims of gas attacks.

'Fortunately for the region, the anticipated casualties never materialised and within six months Booth Hall reverted back to caring for sick children,' Mr Tate said. 'The inscription on Humphrey Booth's headstone reads "Love his memory, imitate his devotion", and I think you will all agree that is an excellent standard to aspire to.'

I felt quite emotional as the coach pulled into Booth Hall. It was a privilege to be a part of the NHS, continuing the good work of the likes of Humphrey Booth, and I was eager to learn about caring for children. I imagined it would be a worthwhile and rewarding branch of nursing, looking after little ones and then returning them, fit and well, back to the bosom of their family. Maybe I might think about being a children's nurse in the future?

It was windy as we walked across the car park to the hospital entrance, where a smiling but straight-backed Matron stood resplendent in a thick cape, arms held wide and welcoming like a priest on a pulpit addressing the congregation.

'Welcome to Booth Hall,' she enunciated with immense pride. 'My staff and I are very pleased to have the opportunity to show off our fine hospital. I hope the visit will serve as an inspiration for you all, girls.'

I caught a glimpse of Linda, who was trying hard to suppress a giggle. 'What?' I whispered.

'Mr Tate,' she said, flicking her eyes over my shoulder.

I turned and saw our tutor grappling unceremoniously with his comb-over, which had become unstuck and was flapping wildly in the breeze, revealing his bald, shiny scalp in all its glory. The escaped hair must have been at least a foot long in full flight.

'Linda, you are awful,' I said. 'Poor Mr Tate!'

We were taken on a whistle-stop tour of several wards and day rooms, which I was heartened to note had colourful bedclothes and curtains and bright pictures on the walls. Children wrapped in dressing gowns and slippers sat quietly with nurses, playing with wooden farmyard animals and train sets. I'd like to do that, I thought.

Our final stop was the burns unit. The smell and stiflingly high temperature hit me as soon as we stepped through the door, and my head immediately started to spin. In here, children were undressed save for their underwear and bandages wrapped around legs, arms, torsos and heads. There was a sickly-sweet smell of flesh mixed together with a petrol-like odour.

Sister Pattinson, who was in charge of the burns unit, patiently started explaining how burns were dressed with open-weave gauze impregnated with Vaseline, which was designed to stop it sticking. I thought how cool and composed she appeared – or was that just in comparison to me? By the time Sister Pattinson got up to the bit about placing the gauze very delicately over the wound so as not to cause more damage to the raw flesh, I was feeling hot and flustered. I was fainting, in fact, and I couldn't stop myself.

I remember hearing the scraping of chair legs and the words: 'Put your head between your legs, Nurse Lawton,' as the ward began to swirl around me. Then I blacked out.

'Never mind, Linda. Happens to the best of us,' Lesley Bennyon told me back at the MRI the following evening, when we signed in for a night shift together.

'I just felt so stupid,' I said. 'What must the children have thought? They are such brave little souls, and there's me, with nothing wrong, collapsing like that in front of them.'

'Put it behind you,' Lesley advised. 'Onwards and upwards! Come on, let's see what's in store tonight.'

Glancing down the ward, I noticed that Mrs Pearlman was fast asleep, which was unusual at the start of a night shift. The night sister had not yet given me my orders, so I walked over to Mrs Pearlman to check on her. She was very still and very quiet, and her black hair had fallen messily across her face. Strands of it were lying across her nose and mouth, and as I got closer I held my breath. Her hair was as still as she was. There was no breath coming from either her nose or her mouth.

I reached for her wrist. There was no pulse, and my own heartbeat quickened, as if to compensate. I smoothed her hair neatly off her face, and pulled the curtain slowly around her bed.

'Lesley,' I said, tears starting to well in my eyes. 'Mrs Pearlman is dead.'

Half an hour later, Lesley and I were tasked with the job of laying out Mrs Pearlman's body. Lesley was an old hand at this by now, but it was my first time and I didn't mind admitting I was a little frightened.

'I don't know what to expect at all,' I told Lesley. 'I've never seen a dead body before, let alone touched one.'

'We'll work together,' Lesley said. 'It's not half as bad as you might think.'

I nodded, silently asking God to help me in my job, and to take good care of Mrs Pearlman.

'She was a very good lady,' I said, telling myself she had lived to a ripe old age and appeared to have died in her sleep, which was a blessing. I guessed that Mrs Pearlman might have anticipated her death, and that is why she'd wanted to give me her gold watch. She was preparing to leave. 'She deserves the best possible care. Please, God, help me to work well, and please may she rest in peace,' I said silently.

Lesley had fetched a trolley upon which she had placed a basin of water, some cloths, cotton wool, bandages and fresh white sheets. There was also a label attached to a piece of string.

'First we have to wash her,' Lesley said quietly, dipping the cotton wool in the water and setting to work, delicately wiping

Mrs Pearlman's face. There were some faint smudges of mascara below the old lady's eyes and some spittle around her mouth, which Lesley tenderly removed.

'There we are,' Lesley said brightly. It was almost as if Mrs Pearlman were still alive and Lesley was chatting to her as she gave her a bed bath.

For a moment I had to remind myself that Mrs Pearlman was very much dead. I stared at her face and could scarcely believe she could no longer talk or smile, because she looked for all the world as if she were in a deep sleep and might wake up at any moment.

Lesley caught my eye. 'Let's pop her teeth back in, shall we?' she said, reaching for Mrs Pearlman's dentures.

I'd been taught the theory of laying out a patient in school, but putting it into practice was another thing entirely.

Lesley opened Mrs Pearlman's mouth gently and inserted the false teeth effortlessly, before flashing me a sympathetic smile. 'There now, she looks better already,' she said. 'Once, I had to lay out a man whose body was cold and rigor mortis had started to set in. It took the strength of two of us to prise open his jaw and squeeze his dentures back in place!'

I smiled gamely, and Lesley kept talking. 'How about we pop a little label on her toe?'

Lesley picked up the brown label upon which she wrote 'Moran Pearlman' and her dates of birth and death. I calculated she had been seventy-six years of age, and was glad she had lived a long life. 'Here, Linda, this needs tying around her big toe,' Lesley said, placing the label in my hand and giving me a nudge of encouragement as I got to work.

Then I watched as Lesley set about packing Mrs Pearlman's body. 'It's not a pleasant job, but honestly, it gets easier each time,' Lesley soothed. 'I was exactly the same as you this time last year – worse, probably!'

I admired Lesley. She somehow managed to keep the atmosphere light yet respectful as she demonstrated first how to bandage around the jaw to keep the mouth closed, and then how to insert cotton wool into the nose and ears to stop any bodily fluids leaking out.

As we gently turned Mrs Pearlman over to wash her back, the old lady let out a slow sigh as her lungs expelled her last breath. Even though I'd been told about this in school, it still took me by surprise, and my hands shot to my mouth.

'Eerie, isn't it?' Lesley said as she continued her work.

All that remained was to wrap Mrs Pearlman's body in a paper shroud and sheets and place a large white label around her legs, which Lesley also wrote her name on. We had just finished the job and were about to call the mortuary porters when a sister stuck her head around the curtain and groaned.

'The Rabbi is on his way!' she said crossly. 'Honestly, Lesley, you ought to know better.'

Lesley's face fell, and she immediately set about unwinding the sheets from Mrs Pearlman's body. I looked at her in confusion.

'It's because she's Jewish,' Lesley hissed, shaking her head and furrowing her brow. 'And Sister is right. I really ought to know better. The Rabbi always visits and says prayers before the body is wrapped up and taken to the morgue. Step outside, Linda. Please detain the Rabbi a moment if he turns up before I'm done unwrapping her.'

Later, after two porters wheeled Mrs Pearlman's body away in what looked like a metal coffin upon a trolley, I felt a sob in my throat. Tears sprang to my eyes, which I couldn't stop from dripping down my cheeks.

'Have a good cry,' Lesley said. 'You wouldn't be human if you didn't. I used to cry every time.'

'H-h-how did you stop?' I asked, accepting a hankie and blowing my nose quietly into it.

'There's no special trick, but thinking about how terrible you look with puffy eyes helps – especially if you think of the handsome house doctors I've spotted recently! Come on, let's sneak ourselves a cup of tea before we go back on the ward.'

A few days later I relayed the story of my first 'laying out' to Graham in intricate detail, complete with fresh tears, which flooded rather than dripped this time.

'People are dying,' I bawled. 'This is harder than I thought.' Sharing the experience diluted the awfulness a little, and as always Graham was a willing shoulder to cry on.

'It's all good experience for you,' he said kindly. 'Your friend is right, I'm sure. It can only get easier.'

He had taken me to one of our favourite little snack bars on Oxford Road. As I sipped a Coca-Cola and ate a Wagon Wheel, I dried my tears and looked at Graham lovingly. I couldn't imagine life without him. I didn't want to go back to the nurses' home on my own, and I laid my head on his shoulder and sobbed.

The following evening, after my shift, I telephoned Graham from the payphone along the corridor of the nurses' home. Feeding four penny coins into the slot, pressing 'A' when I got the connection and hearing his voice saying 'Ashton 4319' had become something of a ritual.

'I'm sorry about last night,' I said. I was so tired I had fallen asleep on his shoulder in the snack bar. He had gently roused me and driven me back to the nurses' home in time for the 11 p.m. curfew. I couldn't thank him enough. Getting a telling off from the home sister on top of everything else would have been too much to bear.

Alone in my room, I studied myself in the mirror properly for the first time in weeks and was shocked by what I saw. There were thick black rings under my eyes and my uniform was sagging around my bust and hips. I'd been a size eight when I started at the MRI and I could see I'd lost weight. Even my hair looked thinner as it hung limply around my ears.

I collapsed into bed and closed my eyes as tightly as possible, telling myself a good night's sleep was what I needed. Through the darkness, two images of Mrs Pearlman's face appeared and began to completely occupy the blackness in my head. First I saw her sitting up in bed, smiling at me, and then I saw her lying cold and still on the morgue trolley. I snapped my eyes open and tried to get her face out of my mind, but each time I closed my eyes, there she was again.

What was I doing to myself in this place? I'm sure I looked worse than some of the patients, and once again I found myself questioning my choice of career, searching for reasons to stay but finding reasons to leave.

Seeing Lesley's smiling face the next morning helped to bring back my smile. She'd been on night duty and was about to clock off.

'You missed a right kerfuffle last night,' she told me. 'We had a tramp brought in, poor old devil. Police called an ambulance after finding him in an alleyway behind Piccadilly Station. We couldn't make out if he was drunk or just delirious. He's in that side room on the end.'

Lesley was holding a tray containing several sputum jars – little pots given to the patients to spit mucus into, so the contents could be taken to the laboratory for testing. She looked perfectly at ease with her revolting wares, and she laughed when she saw me shudder.

'Come on, Linda,' she said. 'Chin up. Now you've laid out a body you've seen it all. There's no going back. If you can do that, nothing else can rattle you!'

I nodded reluctantly. 'Come with me while I check on our poor old tramp before I go,' she said, linking her arm through mine. 'I'm afraid he still doesn't smell too good, despite having had a bed bath and some fresh clothes. No doubt he'll be glad of a cup of tea when the trolley comes round in a bit …'

We entered the side room and both shrieked in unison. Tiny black dots were crawling all over the tramp's pillow and counterpane, but the old man was completely motionless.

'Stay there,' Lesley said, leaving me rooted in the doorway as she stepped up to the bed and lifted his limp arm to test his pulse. I could tell he'd passed away, which didn't appear to surprise Lesley.

'I've seen this before,' she told me solemnly, staring at the pillow. 'It's lice, hundreds of them by the looks of it, leaving his body as it starts to go cold.'

I was speechless.

'There's two beds need making on the ward,' Lesley said swiftly. 'Go quickly and busy yourself while I talk to Sister.'

I thanked Lesley profusely for letting me go.

'Don't mention it,' she said. 'It just goes to show: I guess you can never presume you've seen it all in nursing. Sorry you had to see this, so soon after Mrs Pearlman.'

* * *

Miss Morgan retired at the end of my first year as a student nurse, and a new matron called Miss Bell arrived. She too had an ample bosom, which seemed to be a prerequisite for the job, but I was pleased to see that she also had a refreshingly sunny smile. Her dark chestnut hair was as glossy as fresh conkers, and I was quietly impressed by her each time I saw her patrolling the wards. I thought how glamorous she looked compared to me, even though I was still a teenager and she must have been a middle-aged woman.

'Matron's coming!' someone would caution with unnerving regularity. With Miss Morgan I'd been inclined to hide my head in a locker or dart into the linen cupboard and wish her far away, but when Miss Bell appeared I always wanted to catch a glimpse of her, and I didn't feel the need to hide. She was immaculately presented and exuded confidence and charm. Like Sister Barnes, she made me aspire to be like her. 'You can do it,' I told myself time and time again. I could be like them if I kept working hard, looking after myself and trying my best. I didn't have ambitions to be a matron or even a sister, as those jobs seemed a million miles away from me, but I wanted to be the best nurse possible.

'I'd like to ask your father for your hand in marriage,' Graham announced one evening. We were sitting in an unglamorous café on Deansgate, warming our hands on mugs of hot chocolate.

I giggled, embarrassed. Graham had said many times 'When we get married ...' and in my heart I had known for a long time that he was 'the one' and we would no doubt settle down together eventually. I hadn't been expecting this formal proposal right now, though, not while I had two more years as a student ahead of me. Nevertheless, I was thrilled.

'OK!' I grinned, adding without hesitation: 'I'd like that very much.'

A few weeks later Graham took me to a jewellery shop called Wilds in Ashton. We looked at engagement rings in the window, feeling terribly excited and grown up, before going round to my parents' for our tea.

'You go upstairs, out the way, after we've finished eating,' Graham plotted nervously. 'I'll ask your dad when your mum takes the pots into the kitchen.'

Graham's plan worked like a dream, and my father readily agreed to the marriage, as I was sure he would. Even though I was so young – still just nineteen years old – both my parents were delighted at the news. In those days it wasn't unusual to get engaged at that age.

'We'll have an engagement party,' Mum said when we all gathered in the lounge. 'Ooh Linda, how exciting!'

It was agreed we'd get Christmas out of the way and hold the party early the next year. That would give Graham time to save up to buy a second-hand solitaire ring that had caught my eye at Wilds.

'I'm so pleased for you,' Mum said. 'I'll make some lovely mushroom vol-au-vents and salmon and cucumber finger rolls and trifle for the party and, oh, let me see now, what else? We could do Snowballs and Pomagne cider and …'

We all started to laugh. 'Listen to me!' Mum chuckled. 'I want it to be an occasion to remember. I'm so proud of you, Linda love.'

Dad just sat in his chair smiling, and Graham was grinning from ear to ear. I wanted to keep on making them proud, each one of them.

From that day on, I often thought of their three delighted faces when I pulled on my nurse's uniform and got on with my training. I was doing the right thing as a dutiful daughter and committed wife-to-be. I wanted to make them all so very proud of me, always.

Chapter Five

*'I have come to tender my
resignation, Matron'*

A few months into my second year, around February 1968, I was assigned to a medical ward for patients with kidney problems. I knew very little about kidney failure but I was excited when I was shown the special room that housed the dialysis equipment. To me, it looked like a scene from the film *The Time Machine*, based on the book by H.G. Wells. I remembered seeing posters around town advertising it, showing a weird and wonderful contraption that took you to another world.

Here I felt as if I'd stepped into a science-fiction scene myself, but there wasn't just one strange, metal machine before me – the whole room was full of them. Patients would spend a whole day in the dialysis room, I was told, as the biggest of the grey machines whirled and clicked and pumped, removing waste from their blood because their own kidneys couldn't do the job for them.

I met two very special people on the renal ward. The first was Ronald Buxton, who was thirty-five years old with two children called Bobby and Sandra. He proudly showed me pictures of his son and daughter, telling me they were aged five and seven and the 'loveliest kids in the world'. Bobby supported Manchester United and fancied himself as the next Bobby

Charlton, while Sandra had won trophies for tap dancing and wanted to perform on *Top of the Pops* when she grew up. I met the children once and they were as adorable as I'd imagined, kissing their daddy and presenting him with home-made get well cards they had coloured in carefully.

Ronald's wife, Chrissie, was as quiet as a mouse. She visited every day, topping up her husband's supply of his favourite Fig Roll biscuits and sitting quietly and holding his hand. Ronald was waiting for a new kidney, and on each visit Chrissie would ask hopefully, 'Is there any news, Ron?'

'Not yet, love,' he would say. 'Not yet.'

My heart would ache for them. The same scene played out for six or seven weeks of my two-month placement.

The other patient I grew attached to was Heather Read. She was twenty-eight years old and had long golden hair, which she would always ask me to brush before her husband visited. 'I want to look nice for him, Nurse,' she would say. 'Do I look pretty, Nurse, do I? I want to look my best for him.'

Her husband David lived in Wales and they had two very young children. He couldn't visit every day, but when he did he always brought his wife a present. As a result, Heather had a beautiful collection of silky nightgowns and some wonderful make-up. She was delighted when he brought in some Max Factor Pancake foundation, which she used to disguise her yellow pallor, and she squealed excitedly when he turned up one day with a Mary Quant blue eyeshadow and jet black eyeliner, which she used to copy the looks of models like Jean Shrimpton and Twiggy.

The first to die was Ronald. I knew he was slipping away, but I wasn't prepared for the truly tragic scene that greeted me one evening. Chrissie had been at his bedside when he passed away, but she couldn't accept he had gone. When I arrived for the night shift she was still shaking his lifeless body and imploring him: 'Please don't leave me, Ron! We need you here with us. Please, Ron, don't leave me! Please don't leave me!'

'She's been in with him for quite a while,' Jennifer, a third-year student, told me sadly. 'I've never heard her say so much in all the time she's been coming in. We shall have to intervene shortly. I've talked to Sister.'

Coaxing Mrs Buxton away from her husband's body was heartbreaking. When I escaped the ward for my meal break later, I rushed off alone to an empty side room so I could sob until my eyeballs ached.

'Dear God, do you really exist?' I asked silently, looking through a window and up at the starry night sky as I crossed the walkway and headed to the canteen. 'If you do, please can you hold my hand?'

I imagined God took hold of my hand and helped me wipe away my tears, but it didn't help. I still felt utterly devastated, and I was glad when I spotted Janice sitting alone at a table for two. Perhaps having a chat with her would cheer me up.

Janice had her head down and was swirling a blob of raspberry jam absent-mindedly into a bowl of steaming semolina.

'How are you?' I asked.

We both watched the pudding turn pink as Janice said miserably, 'Fed up to the back teeth.' She recited a catalogue of woes and told me she had decided to quit. 'I handed in my notice to Miss Bell this morning and I am going in two weeks' time. I can't take it any more, but I have to work my notice.'

'What will you do?' I asked, feeling forlorn.

'Don't know yet,' she replied. 'Anything that doesn't involve blood and guts and death will suit me fine.'

I didn't bother telling her about Ronald. She didn't look as if she could cope with any more depressing news. We were about eighteen months into our training by now – practically halfway through, in fact – and Janice would be leaving with nothing.

'You must have a plan?' I asked.

'I'll be fine,' she said convincingly. 'Getting out of here will be the best thing I ever did. This isn't the life for me, not at all. I've known for a long while, so the brave thing now is to quit and do something I'm better suited to.'

I was very sorry to hear Janice's news. Even though we had quite different personalities, our shared experiences had made us good friends. I would miss her, and for her sake I hoped she was making the right decision. Somehow I felt she was. The fun-loving, exuberant Janice I had first met hadn't been evident for quite some time, and I realised nursing had been making her unhappy, so it was best to go.

Later that same week, I arrived for another night shift to find Heather's bed occupied by an elderly male patient.

'We lost her yesterday,' Jennifer said, giving me a little hug. 'Her husband left you this.' She handed me a beautifully packaged gift, which I stared at. 'He said to say thank you for everything you did, and he wants you to have this to remember Heather by.'

I wanted to open it in private but Jennifer was looking at me expectantly, so I untied the pink velvet ribbon and carefully opened the pretty tissue-paper parcel. Inside there was a small, wooden-handled hairbrush and a note that said: 'Thank you for caring for my beautiful wife. I will always remember how pretty she looked in hospital.'

Unlike with Mrs Pearlman's gold watch, I would not need to ask for permission to keep this gift. It had not been given to me by a patient and it was not a valuable item in monetary terms, but to me it was worth a great deal and I would treasure it.

I tucked it in my pocket and felt choked, as if the breath had been sucked out of my throat, but I didn't cry. I wanted to sob and wail for Heather, but I couldn't. I felt numb with shock and grief. My throat and eyes were as dry as bones. I was exhausted and wrung out. In that moment I decided I couldn't go on either. I would quit, just like Janice, and in two weeks' time I'd be out of there too.

Alone in my room, I composed a brief letter of resignation addressed to Miss Bell, requesting that I be released from my training and explaining briefly that I was struggling to cope and finding it too tough to continue.

The next day I made an appointment with Miss Bell so I could hand-deliver the letter, and if I was forced to explain myself further I intended to tell her I had decided to pursue a career as a nursery nurse instead. I didn't know how I would go about this, but I was convinced that working with children who weren't ill would be a perfect joy compared to nursing, and the thought of it filled me with relief.

I couldn't bring myself to tell Graham what I planned because I knew he would try to talk me out of it, and I had made up my mind. Nor did I tell Nessa, Anne, Jo or Linda, as I knew it would make me feel a failure compared to them. I didn't want a fuss; I just desperately wanted to go home and start again.

Mum would understand eventually, I reasoned. She'd thrown a wonderful engagement party for Graham and me just a few weeks earlier, to coincide with my twentieth birthday in March 1968. As promised, she laid on an impressive spread which included potted salmon finger rolls, cheese and pineapple cubes on sticks, warm vol-au-vents topped with sliced cucumber and presented on doilies, fruit cocktail made with tinned peaches and glacé cherries, plus her signature sherry trifle, topped generously with grated chocolate.

'Georgy Girl' by The Seekers played on the record player in the corner as Graham and I cut our iced fruit cake, which had been lovingly baked by my father. Dad took a few photographs on his new Kodak Instamatic camera, and I still have one or two today. They show me posing happily beside Graham and the sets of crockery and glassware we received as engagement presents. I'm dressed in a long-sleeved black mini dress with little white spots, which has a Peter Pan collar and a row of tiny buttons down the front. When the assembled guests all clapped noisily to toast our happiness, I remember it made the needle on the record jump and Mum put on something by Manfred Mann instead.

After everybody had left and we were clearing up, Mum told me that what she wanted, more than anything, was for me to be happy. She was talking about my married life, of course, but as I grappled with my resignation letter I played with my mother's words in my mind. She would be dreadfully disappointed, but I convinced myself she would ultimately support my decision to quit. She wouldn't want me to be miserable in my work, and nor would my father. They would understand, once they had got over the inevitable shock, and it wouldn't be long before I got myself on a new course, hopefully nursery nursing, and started afresh.

I was trembling when Miss Bell summoned me into her office. 'How can I help you, Nurse Lawton?' she beamed, signalling for me to sit down in front of her desk as she eyed the letter in my hand with astute caution.

'I have come to tender my resignation, Matron,' I said meekly. 'Here is my letter.'

Miss Bell took the letter from me, arched a silky eyebrow and asked, 'May I know the reason?'

Her tone of voice showed no reaction to my dramatic news, and I felt my pulse pounding.

'I don't think nursing is the career for me,' I said apologetically. My voice was wobbling and I was squeezing my hands together on my lap to stop them shaking.

'I see. Please wait here. I just have to slip out.'

With that, Miss Bell swished past me rather majestically, clutching the letter to her bosom.

As the clip-clop of her heels grew fainter, my heartbeat drummed louder. I wanted to run in the opposite direction down the corridor but I sat still, obediently waiting for Miss Bell to get back.

I felt incredibly uncomfortable, not knowing what she might say or do on her return. There was a ticking clock sitting on her desk, and a black telephone. How long would she be? What if the telephone rang? My legs started to jangle. I clenched my toes inside my shoes and tried to anchor my heels firmly onto the floor. I was absolutely terrified, and I sat like that for a full twelve minutes before Miss Bell reappeared.

She was smiling, thank goodness.

'You have struggled at times, Nurse Lawton, haven't you?' she said kindly.

I nodded.

'I do understand. Lots of girls find it very difficult, particularly here at the MRI, where our standards are so exacting.'

I wanted to cry, but I didn't.

Miss Bell was still holding my letter, which she now raised aloft. 'However, I am not just going to accept this,' she said, before folding it briskly in two and depositing it in her desk drawer. 'I am going to send you to St Mary's Maternity Hospital in the centre of town for three months. You will continue to live here. You will have breakfast here each morning and then a taxi will pick you up at 7.30 a.m. sharp and take you to St Mary's. You will have your tea there and you will wear the same uniform, but you must not wear your apron in the taxi. Let's give it a try, shall we?'

I nodded gratefully. I wanted to get out of Miss Bell's office as quickly as possible, and I felt a wave of relief as I realised that although she had not accepted my resignation she had handed me a ticket out of the MRI.

'Go and see Mr Tate now, please. He is expecting you.'

Miss Bell did not expand on why she thought maternity nursing might be the way forward for me, and I am sure she had no idea I had an interest in nursery nursing. To this day, I believe she simply followed her instincts – and how sharp they were!

She must have conferred with Mr Tate during the period when she left me alone in her room because he already knew about my new placement and made a point of wishing me luck. It was very kind of him to help facilitate this opportunity and I thanked him profusely.

Maternity meant babies. How lovely! That could be even better than working with small children, I thought optimistically. I pictured pretty babies gurgling and sleeping peacefully while I made up bottles and fetched their tired but radiant mothers a freshly brewed cup of tea. I had no experience of babies whatsoever – had never even picked one up – but I was suddenly delighted at the prospect. I knew it had to be far better than looking after people who were ill.

My first taxi journey to St Mary's, in April 1968, was quite a thrill. There were three other girls with me, none of whom I knew personally but all of whom seemed equally as excited as me to be going on secondment to St Mary's. I'd only ever ridden in a taxi on a handful of occasions and I felt quite important, being transported along Oxford Road in a shiny black cab, wearing my thick green cloak over my uniform.

I had been told many times that MRI nurses had a reputation for being a 'cut above the rest' and I really felt it now. For the first time I fully understood why Sister Mary Francis had insisted that she only wanted her girls to go to the very best hospital, and I felt extremely proud to wear my uniform in public. I was glad I hadn't quit. I was taking on a new challenge, and I hoped and prayed I would enjoy it a great deal. Surely I would be better suited to dealing with birth than illness?

In the morning rush hour it was about a twenty-minute taxi ride along Oxford Road, which became Oxford Street as you approached the heart of the city. I knew the drive well, as when I went into town shopping with the girls we would take the trolley bus along the same route. Sometimes the electric-powered bus would lose its connection with the cable above and the conductor would have to get off and use a long pole to reconnect it to the electric wire running overhead. The trolley bus stopped every few minutes to pick people up, or so it seemed, and no sooner had you breathed a sigh of relief at a throng of passengers disembarking than another crowd pushed on.

The taxi was luxurious by comparison. I looked out the window at the office workers walking briskly in the early spring sunshine. The men wore wide-collared shirts and knitted ties, and the women were mostly dressed in mini skirts and kitten heels, or draped in voluminous pastel-coloured macs, secured at the neck with a fancy brooch or neatly tied scarf. There was quite a bit of traffic on the roads at this hour of the morning. Everyone was going somewhere, and there was a definite buzz in the air.

The cab's engine hummed as we pulled up outside St Mary's. The splendid-looking red-brick hospital stood next to the Ritz and opposite the Palace Theatre, on the corner of Oxford Street. All of the buildings looked unfamiliar in the morning light, and I felt a tingle of excitement at the prospect of exploring my new surroundings. I was entering unfamiliar territory all over again, yet I sensed this was going to be much more manageable than the MRI. It might even be fun.

I'd been asked to report on arrival to the office of Mrs Ingham, the senior obstetric nursing tutor at St Mary's. I knew nothing about her, except that Miss Bell had spoken to her about me.

As I stepped inside the maternity hospital for the first time, I was struck by how bright and cheerful it felt for such an old building. Beams of light were streaming in through the windows, of which there were many, and there was a low but distinctive chorus in the air of babies snuffling and crying, and mothers and midwives soothing and shushing.

'Welcome to St Mary's,' Mrs Ingham said warmly when I entered her office. She smiled from ear to ear, and I found myself smiling back. 'I've heard some very good things about you, Nurse Lawton. It sounds to me as if you have the makings of a very good nurse, perhaps even an obstetrics nurse, and I am here to help you on your way.'

I felt instantly at ease with Mrs Ingham. She was middle-aged with grey hair and had the demeanour of a kindly older aunt. She appeared rather no-nonsense on the surface but, as I later found out, she had a heart as soft as putty.

'I have assigned you to one of the postnatal wards for normal deliveries,' she explained. 'You are here principally to observe, but you will learn how to bathe and swaddle the newborns, feed and change them and generally care for their mothers during their stay with us.'

It sounded easy, though I had never made up a bottle or pinned a nappy in my life. From my experience at the MRI, however, I expected that caring for the mothers and newborns would mean a lot more than making tea, mopping brows and rocking babies to sleep. Nevertheless I felt sure it would be much more pleasant dealing with new life than coping with sickness and death.

'Don't worry, you won't be asked to do anything you don't feel able to do,' Mrs Ingham said, as if she had just read my mind. 'I'm sure you'll prove to be a very useful little helper.'

'I hope so,' I said.

'That's a good girl,' Mrs Ingham replied. 'Let's get started, shall we?'

She took me to a ward that occupied a corner of the building, and had high windows on three sides. The walls were painted bright white and laser-like sunbeams pierced the air overhead. I blinked and felt a smile twitching at the corners of my lips. There was a lovely smell of warm milk and talcum powder.

Beds lined all three walls, and each bed had a cot standing beside it. I was interested to see the cots were like little cloth hammocks fixed between two metal stands. Some babies were asleep in the cots while others were being fed or changed. At a glance it was impossible to tell which were boys and which were girls, as each baby was dressed in an identical white cotton nightie, fastened with three little bows up the back.

There was so much to take in, I didn't know what to look at first, or where each of the noises was coming from. Some babies were griping while others squeaked and cried. One or two mums were talking animatedly. Others sat quietly, bottle-feeding their babies, while a few dozed and snored.

Four midwives were on the ward. One was rocking a grizzly baby in her arms as she sat beside a sleeping mother, and another was distributing glass bottles, filled with baby milk and topped with rubber teats, to the end of each bed. A third midwife was patiently demonstrating how to fold a cloth nappy correctly and insert the pins without 'using baby's bottom as a pin cushion', and a fourth was pushing a trolley laden with cot linen and cotton wool.

Each midwife looked calm and approachable. Their skirts were full and long and their substantial aprons were strapped and starched and pinned neatly, though somehow they didn't look quite as smart as the MRI nurses. Their image appealed to me a great deal. It was hard to put your finger on it, but the midwives looked less starchy and more modern than the nurses at the MRI. Each had a shiny fob watch attached to her breast pocket, which stood proud of the apron and looked for all the world like a well-deserved medal of honour.

Mrs Ingham introduced me to a ward sister called Sister Rose. 'I'm very pleased to welcome you, Nurse Lawton,' she said genuinely. 'Come into my office and I will run through a few basics. We're extremely glad to have an extra pair of hands on the ward.'

Sister Rose was laid back compared to most of the sisters I had encountered at the MRI. She made the routine on her ward sound very simple. Ladies who had just delivered and had no complications came to this postnatal ward. They would be required to stay in bed for six hours, strictly without exception, to give their uterus the chance to contract and settle after giving birth. It would be my job to take each lady a bedpan if she required one in that time, and to provide her with bottles of milk, terry nappies and pins and cotton wool for her baby.

'We wake the babies routinely to feed them every four hours,' Sister Rose explained. 'Babies must be encouraged to feed even if they don't appear hungry. A strict routine is important, and no bottles are to be distributed between regular feed times.'

Newborn babies, I learned, were lifted away from the mother immediately after they were born. New mothers only held their baby briefly for the first time after the midwife had weighed and dressed the infant, wiped its face and head if need be and swaddled it snugly. Each baby was then taken away to the nursery and bathed by the midwife before finally being handed to the mother. In those days, the bonding and subsequent breastfeeding benefits of immediate skin-to-skin contact for mother and baby were yet to be discovered.

'When they are in their cots, we swaddle them and lay the babies to sleep on their tummies,' Sister Rose explained. 'This helps them to sleep soundly.'

Later research would recommend laying babies on their backs and not swaddling them too tightly to reduce the risk of overheating and even cot death, but that was many years in the future.

I was also told that the women on this ward were routinely given a drug called Stilboestrol to suppress lactation, as it was nowhere near as fashionable to breastfeed as it is today. Some ladies wished to drink dissolved Epsom salts, believing they helped the body expel fluid which they hoped would further reduce the milk levels in the breasts.

'In my opinion, this is an old wives' tale,' Sister Rose told me, rolling her eyes playfully, 'but there is no evidence to suggest Epsom salts are in any way detrimental to a new mother, so our ladies are allowed to take them if they wish.' She added that patients who could not get out of bed might require help with 'douching' and that most ladies stayed in hospital until their baby was six days old.

'Do you have any questions?' she asked, finally.

I told her that I didn't have any questions just yet, although the truth was I had plenty. What was 'douching' and, more importantly, would I be allowed to see a baby being born? The mechanics of giving birth fascinated me. My mother had never disclosed any details of how the magical process worked, and I had never dared to ask. Mum got flustered when she had to tell me about periods, and after she had provided me with a sanitary belt and towels in my early teens we never spoke of such matters again. I'd studied biology, of course, and had a textbook understanding of reproduction and birth, but how a real-life baby emerged into the world from its mother's womb was still a mystery to me.

At the end of the day I was delighted to spill out onto Oxford Street and hear the sound of music bubbling under the door of the Ritz. It had a reputation as one of the smartest dance halls in town and was far too expensive for a student like me, but I enjoyed being tantalisingly close to where it was 'happening'.

I liked to listen to Radio Luxemburg whenever I could, and the DJs were forever reminding listeners that we lived in the 'Swinging Sixties'. Here, in the heart of Manchester, I could feel the swing. It probably wasn't anything like as exciting as in the heart of London, but I could certainly feel the beat. The evening air smelled of fish and chips and beer, and I inhaled deeply. If it weren't for the fact I was clad in my nurse's uniform, I'd have swung my hips before I skipped into the taxi that shuttled me back to the MRI.

When I got back to the nurses' home after my first day at St Mary's, I had a rare pow-wow with Nessa, Jo, Anne and Linda. Unusually, we happened to be on our way in at the same time, each one of us desperate for a bath and bed, but we agreed to snatch ten minutes together in the communal lounge area. It was drab in that room and there was often a home sister nosing around so we usually avoided it, but that evening we were too tired to care so we all slumped into the nearest available threadbare armchairs.

'How's the baby hospital?' Linda asked me. 'Delivered any yet?'

'Course not!' I laughed. 'I haven't even picked a baby up yet, let alone delivered one! I think I'm going to like it, though. It feels like a breath of fresh air. It's like stepping out of a long, cold winter into spring after being here at the MRI.'

'Wow!' Jo said. 'Sounds like someone's found her vocation!'

'Perhaps,' I smiled, enjoying the thought. I definitely had a good vibe about the place, there was no doubt about it.

Jo then regaled us with a hilarious tale of how she was caught unawares by two dishy house doctors, Frank and Tom, who discovered it had been her birthday the week before. As she finished her night shift and walked down an empty corridor they pounced out of a broom cupboard with a couple of sheets, in which they swiftly wrapped her up.

'My heart was pounding!' she said.

'Bet it was,' Linda said, giving a cheeky wink. 'Which one do you fancy more – Frank or Tom?'

'Well, they're both gorgeous but I'd never get involved with a house doctor,' she said. 'We all know what they're like: happy to flirt but underneath it all they're as worn out as old men and too tired to do anything!' Seemingly as an afterthought, she added: 'Besides, you know I have a boyfriend, you rotten lot.'

After picking Jo up in the sheet, the cheeky young doctors pushed her into a wheelchair, whizzed her to a bathroom and dunked her in a bath of cold water. It was not an uncommon prank at the MRI, we learned.

'I had to laugh,' Jo said. 'But I wanted to belt the pair of them. My uniform was still damp the next morning.'

'Talking of uniform …' Linda chuckled. 'Guess who's been a naughty girl?'

'You!' we all chimed. Linda had been heading for trouble since a few weeks earlier she'd finally cracked and asked Cynthia Weaver for advice on how to shorten the hem of her dress.

'Honestly, it was only just on the knee,' Linda hooted. 'Thank God Miss Morgan has gone. Miss Bell still gave me a pretty tough telling off, but she didn't pull the stitches out in the middle of the corridor as old Miss Morgan would have done.'

'I'll be keeping my eye on you from now on, Nurse Mochri!'
Linda thrust out her chest in a fine impersonation of Miss Bell,
which made us all laugh.

Nessa expressed her sadness at Janice's departure. She had
been the last to know, it seemed, and never even got the chance
to say goodbye. We all reassured her that it was nothing
personal. Janice had wanted to slip away quietly and none of
us had heard from her since, despite asking her to keep in
touch.

'It seems such a shame to walk away with nothing, not even
friends,' Nessa said. 'When you think of poor Cynthia …
What she wouldn't give to be able to finish the course.'

We all looked at Nessa expectantly. 'What's happened to
Cynthia?' Linda asked.

The pair of us had been with her just a few weeks earlier,
when she taught us how use some clever embroidery to
customise a couple of handbags we picked up at the market.

Nessa had fallen quiet. She had not expected to be the one
to deliver this news and didn't like taking centre stage, but all
eyes were on her.

'Cynthia was diagnosed with a serious heart condition last
week. She has a hole in her heart and needs to have open-heart
surgery. She's being treated on Ward S2.'

We all just gaped. Cynthia was a nurse, not a patient. She
always looked tired, but then again we all did. There had been
nothing to indicate she had such a serious condition, although
I did recall her paying several visits to the sick bay of late.

'Apparently her lips had started to go blue quite a lot, but
she hadn't thought anything of it,' Nessa explained. 'That was,
until she collapsed on a ward at the end of a night shift.
Hopefully we'll be allowed to visit her soon.'

'They can do remarkable things now,' Jo interjected, trying to be positive. 'Look what they did in South Africa.'

Surgeon Christiaan Barnard had carried out the world's first heart transplant just before the previous Christmas. I remembered there was tinsel hanging in the dining room when I discussed it with a group of other nurses. The Pill had become available to unmarried women around the same time, which I recalled had been another subject for debate – one we were rather more animated about, to tell the truth.

As student nurses we may not have been at the cutting edge of medical breakthroughs, but we certainly felt proud to be a small part of such a pioneering profession, and we chewed over such news whenever we got the chance.

Nessa, Jo, Anne, Linda and I all knew that Christiaan Barnard's ground-breaking transplant patient died within weeks of receiving his new heart, but none of us made reference to that fact.

'Poor Cynthia,' said Linda, who had blanched. 'Why do people have to get ill?'

Nobody had an answer, and I knew Linda well enough to realise her question was as much about her mum's cancer as it was about Cynthia. I knew her mum's condition was deteriorating, and that Linda was very worried about her.

I went to bed that night with Linda's words pressing on my mind: why do people have to get ill? It was a question without an answer, and one that made me feel all the more grateful for my placement at St Mary's, where the days were filled with new life rather than sickness and death. Perhaps Jo was right. Perhaps I had found my vocation, working at the maternity hospital. I wasn't quite sure about being an obstetric nurse as I didn't know much about the job at that stage, but I certainly wanted to find out more. I fell asleep looking forward to climbing into the taxi the next day, travelling into the beating heart of the city and taking care of all those tiny little babies and their mums.

Chapter Six

'Nurse Lawton, you have been granted permission to witness a birth if you come quickly'

'I'm happy to see you're working so well here at St Mary's,' Sister Rose said one morning as I reported for duty. She had a small transistor radio on her desk, and I could just make out the DJ announcing the Rolling Stones' new single, 'Jumpin' Jack Flash'. As the record crackled onto the airways I couldn't help tuning in, and I inadvertently tapped my foot in time to the music.

Sister Rose switched off the radio instantly and gave me a stern look, as if to say, 'Let's not be having any of that here.'

'As I was saying,' she went on firmly, 'I want you to know that if you continue in the same vein I shall be giving you an excellent report to take back to the MRI. I believe you have the makings of a very good obstetric nurse.'

I felt myself blush. I hadn't expected such a compliment. I still had more than a year to go before I even qualified as a nurse, let alone made any decisions about my future career. I had been telling myself to take things steadily, take my time and weigh up my options carefully, but my reaction to Sister Rose's compliment made me realise how much this placement meant to me. I was invigorated by her words. I wanted to excel here, because I was starting to believe it was the gateway to my future.

'If you would like to broaden your horizons, I can arrange for you to observe a delivery,' Sister Rose proposed.

'Oh, yes please!' I said enthusiastically. 'I should like that very much.'

'Excellent! Please attend to the milk kitchen this morning, and I will see what I can do.'

I loved the milk kitchen. Making up the feeds made me feel very useful, and even though this seemingly mundane task was assigned to me every day I always took the utmost care in sterilising the bottles and measuring out the powdered milk.

The very first time I held a baby, one of the other midwives showed me how to tilt the bottle at just the right angle so as not to allow the newborn to gulp air. The tiny boy, who was no more than a few hours old, attached his rosebud lips greedily to the teat and sucked contentedly. I was captivated. It was an honour to be feeding a brand new baby, feeling his warmth against me and smelling the sweetness of his delicate head. I had a perfect little life in my hands.

'Makes your heart melt, doesn't it?' the midwife said, seeing the enthralled expression on my face.

'Yes, it does!' I replied. 'That's exactly the right phrase. I could get used to this!'

The milk kitchen was housed in a side room just off the ward, and each day I would boil water in a giant-sized metal kettle while I washed the glass bottles and rinsed out the brown rubber teats that needed to be stretched over the top of them. All the equipment then had to be placed in a cage and lowered into a large metal steriliser unit, which hissed and boiled and spat. Meanwhile, I measured out the boiled water and carefully counted each spoonful of dried milk powder into a large stainless steel jug and mixed it up with a sterilised spoon. Retrieving the bottles was always slightly unnerving, as they had to be hooked out of the steriliser cage with small forceps, taking care to tip out any drops of water, lest they would splatter your uniform or burn your hands.

Pouring the yellow-tinted liquid into the bottles was an exact science. I would typically make up two dozen batches of two-ounce and four-ounce feeds, as that was about as much as the tiny mites could manage in one sitting. I'd been shown how to squeeze a few drips of milk onto the inside of my wrist to check it was not too hot, and once the correct temperature was reached I was able to distribute the bottles around the ward, leaving one at the end of each bed ready for the babies to be woken and fed, always at exactly the same time.

Occasionally, if there were some milk left over, I would hide away in the kitchen and discreetly have a little drink of it myself. I liked the sweet taste, and it helped keep my energy levels up.

'Have you saved enough for my Tommy?' one friendly patient, Rosemary, asked me one day.

'Pardon?' I replied, flustered.

She looked at my mouth and gestured for me to wipe around my lips.

'Oh!' I exclaimed, feeling extremely embarrassed.

'It don't bother me!' she chuckled. 'Don't expect Sister would be best pleased, though!'

I enjoyed chatting to the women. There was something magical about being involved in their lives at such a momentous time. Despite being tired out after giving birth, they were nearly always in good spirits and their shared experience created an open and friendly atmosphere on the ward.

Funnily enough, conversations were hardly ever about babies. The new mothers cooed over them and admired each other's newborns, of course, but the women didn't obsess about potential ailments, pre-school provision and the pros and cons of certain foods as they tend to do today. Instead, they talked about the latest episode of *The Prisoner* or *Coronation Street* they'd seen on telly, swapped crochet patterns for matinée jackets and booties and bickered over whether Tom Jones was more of a dish than Elvis.

When their families visited, proud new dads and excited siblings would stick their noses excitedly into the hammock cot beside the bed, and then the kids would exhaust the mother with a million and one questions. 'Have we got enough tokens off the marmalade to send off for a Golly badge?' 'Where's the new lace for my football?' '*Please* can we get the cornflakes with the toy in the bottom of the packet?'

The only time most married women stayed away from their husbands and children was when they were in hospital after giving birth, and it was touching to see their presence at home was clearly missed.

'Will I be able to wear my roller skates when we take the baby out in the new pram?' or 'Can we make a go-cart out of the old pram?' were questions I heard more than once, along with the old chestnut from the dads: 'Is it OK if Mrs So-and-so takes in our washing, only I can't figure out how the twin tub works …?'

I enjoyed the daily routine on the ward. Once the bottles were made, I might help another midwife with douching the patients, which I learned was simply washing between their legs. I admired the midwives for the way they managed this task so efficiently, never compromising a woman's comfort or dignity. Their skill seemed to strip away any embarrassment I'd imagined such a job might entail.

Next it would be time to change and bathe the babies. The square cloths used to make up the terry nappies arrived in stiff piles from the hospital laundry each morning. They smelled so strongly of Ajax laundry detergent they made my nostrils tingle, but at least there was never any doubt about their cleanliness. They were always pristine and spotless.

I was taught how to gently wash the baby down with warm water and cotton wool and apply a generous coating of zinc and castor oil cream to the bottom to ward off nappy rash, before folding the cloth into a neat nappy.

Little girls, I learned, were best placed in kite-shaped nappies, where you folded the top down and then the side in, while little boys stayed drier in triangle-shaped nappies with more padding at the front. I tried to use the metal safety pins with pink guard covers for girls and save the blue ones for boys, as it was the only way of distinguishing between the sexes once the babies were dressed in their NHS nighties. Nobody brought their own baby clothes into hospital in those days, so it was regulation white cotton nighties all round. Dirty nappies, mercifully, were dumped straight in the wash bin and sent off to be dealt with by the laundry.

It only took me a few weeks to become an expert at bathing babies, and to be able to show new mums how to do it.

'Wish I could take ye home with me, Nurse,' a new mum said to me one day as I gave her a demonstration in the nursery, where we had a special, low porcelain sink for bathing the babies.

Her compliment thrilled me. Inside, I felt like such an amateur, so young and inexperienced, yet somehow I must have looked competent as I gently lowered her wriggling baby into the water, taking care to hold the little girl under her arms and keep her face out of the water.

'You'll be fine,' I reassured the woman. She was probably only a year or two older than me, as most women started their families in their early to mid twenties back then, and I was flattered to see she was hanging on my every word.

'Practice makes perfect. You just need to test the water temperature with your elbow to make sure it is not too hot or too cold, and make sure you have a steady grip on your baby. Here, come and try.'

It was an honour to witness special moments like that. Many of the mums came from the most poverty-stricken areas spread around the city. They wore poor-quality nightdresses, often had a sneaky drag on a cigarette when Sister wasn't looking, and many cussed routinely in their strong Manchester accents. Whatever their background, I found that the vast majority had the manners of a princess. They would thank me kindly for everything I did, tell me I was an angel and beam at me with gratitude when I made my way round the ward checking temperatures and pulses, or delivering mugs of Horlicks before lights out.

I didn't do many night shifts at St Mary's, but I found myself looking forward to being on the ward after dark. Lights out was strictly at 10 p.m., and the night sister would discourage the new mothers from getting up unless they had a very good reason. Usually I was sent into the nursery, where all the babies were taken to give their mothers a chance to sleep soundly. Sometimes I had a baby in my arms and would be rocking one or two others in cribs, using my feet.

'What a racket!' the night sister often exclaimed when the babies were grizzling and fighting sleep. I didn't like to hear them cry, but the noise didn't offend me. I enjoyed cuddling the babies, however noisy they were. I found it very rewarding to soothe them with a gentle 'sh-sh-sh' as their fidgety little bodies and fragile, flailing limbs gradually turned to heavy, sleeping weights in my arms.

It was warm in the nursery, and there was always a pleasant, convivial atmosphere. In the end, I often couldn't hear the crying, I got so used to it. I'd sit and look out the window and watch amorous couples walking arm and arm into the Ritz or the Palace, amusing myself with thoughts of what the future held for them. Would they have babies, and would they look out of the window of St Mary's one day and say, 'Oooh, I remember going to the Ritz back in the spring of 1968 …'?

'Eee, will you look at this funny baby,' the midwives would giggle to each other from time to time. 'Only a mother could love it!'

It was gentle banter to pass the time and lighten the atmosphere, nothing more. The midwives all seemed to enjoy their work, and the chit-chat flowed easily amid the chorus of newborn cries and snuffles.

Once, I heard some older midwives whispering about a 'termination' case. I never joined in conversations like that, as I could tell when they wanted to keep something hush-hush and I didn't want to say the wrong thing. However, I picked up that a young girl without a baby was occupying bed eleven on the ward. She had been sent here to rest following her operation, I gathered, because there was nowhere else for her to go. The curtain was closed tightly around her bed, which was understandable. I thought how terrible it must be for her to hear newborn babies all around, not to mention the proud new mothers chatting happily away to each other.

Abortion was something very new for the midwives to contend with, as it had only recently been legalised and was now offered free on the NHS. The Abortion Act of 1967 came into effect on 27 April 1968, after initially being introduced as a Private Member's Bill by David Steel. I had followed the news with interest as the bill passed through Parliament, not realising how close I would come to the reality of it all. I learned that most women in this situation were cared for on a gynaecology ward at the MRI rather than at the maternity hospital, although a minority had started to trickle through to St Mary's.

'The cut-off points all seem a bit arbitrary,' one midwife lamented. She was referring to the fact that unless there were extreme circumstances abortions were only carried out on the NHS up to fourteen weeks, and yet a foetus was not considered viable until it was twenty-eight weeks old. This meant that if a woman delivered prematurely prior to twenty-eight weeks, doctors and midwives were not encouraged to attempt resuscitation if there were no signs of life.

'I know what you mean,' another, much older, midwife replied. 'I think twenty-eight weeks is about right, but then again we all know how well formed a foetus is just before twenty-eight weeks. It's a tough call deciding when a baby is a baby and not a foetus.'

A low hum of agreement went round the little nursery. I could feel tension in the air and could tell the midwives were not entirely comfortable with this topic. Delivering babies was their role, not this.

'But at least this Act is a step in the right direction,' the older midwife ploughed on. 'It's better to make abortion legal than force these poor girls into back-street clinics. Believe me, I've known some terrible cases. The NHS is much better off picking up the bill for terminations than forking out to put these poor women back together again after they've been butchered.'

The word 'butchered' made me shudder, and I felt very glad that, thanks to the new law, the girl in bed eleven was being cared for by professionals in her time of need, rather than having to go to a back-street clinic.

Even when opinions ran high the midwives didn't appear to judge any of the patients, though one or two seemed to enjoy a good gossip.

'Did you know this poor mite's mum is a prostitute?' I heard one midwife, Veronica, hiss to her colleagues one night.

'Never!' the other midwives replied, looking in alarm at baby Paul, the bonny, mixed-race little boy who was sleeping contentedly in my arms.

When I heard the word prostitute I felt myself go red, and with all eyes pointing in my direction I stuttered, 'Is she from the red-light district?'

In my shock and embarrassment, it was the only thing I could think of to say about prostitutes.

'Seems so,' Veronica shrugged sadly. 'Baby's fine, praise the Lord, even though his mother was suspected of having venereal disease.'

I actually gasped as she said it. I'd read about unspeakable infections like syphilis and gonorrhoea in the new 1968 edition of *Textbook for Midwives* by Margaret F. Myles in the library. I'd been absolutely horrified by the gruesome images and explanations, but never for a moment did I think I'd come across anything like this at St Mary's. I thought it was something that only happened to paupers in a bygone era.

'Nurse Lawton, you have been granted permission to witness a birth if you come quickly,' Sister Rose said, appearing unexpectedly in the doorway.

The nursery fell completely silent at the sight of Sister Rose. Even though she was a very easy-going sister compared to most I had met at the MRI, her rank meant there was an automatic response to her presence. Each midwife straightened her back and there was a rustle of throat-clearing and smoothing down of skirts and aprons. All talk of abortions and prostitutes was well and truly over, and the midwives tilted their heads diligently towards their tiny charges, cooing and shushing gently, as if a switch had been flicked.

Sister Rose's eyes scanned the room approvingly before resting on me once more. 'Follow me!' she ordered. 'You need to come right away.'

I hurriedly handed baby Paul to Veronica, my heart leaping into my mouth as I scuttled after Sister Rose, hanging on her every word.

'This is a third baby and labour has advanced very nicely, without complications. Just stand quietly beside me and watch.'

I nodded, feeling a well of exhilaration rise from my heart and rush to every tingling nerve in my body.

Outside the delivery room was a young man in his mid twenties who was wearing workman's boots and a donkey jacket with leather pads on the elbows. He was alternating between dragging heavily on a cigarette and biting his nicotine-stained nails nervously.

'Look after 'er, won't ye?' he asked as he stepped aside to let us pass.

'Of course we will, Mr Hollingworth!' Sister Rose said reassuringly.

'Thank you kindly, Nurses!' he called after us, saluting us with the hand in which he held his cigarette.

His wife let out a piercing scream as we pushed through the delivery room doors. There was a midwife at the foot of the bed and another one busying herself with the resuscitaire trolley, which was next to a table where a gleaming pair of scales stood. I noted with some surprise that the scales looked like the ones the greengrocer used to weigh turnips and potatoes in Ashton Market.

'Can you give me one last big push, Mrs Hollingworth?' the midwife said in a voice that was somehow both authoritative and gently encouraging. 'You are doing *ever* so well.'

Mrs Hollingworth seemed completely oblivious to our arrival and let out a loud cry of 'Aye, I can do that, Nurse,' before gobbling in air and gripping the sides of the blanket that were draped over her body. She was wearing a thick cotton nightdress with a stand-up collar laced tightly up her neck. Her face was so red and sweaty it looked as if it had been squeezed out of the stiff collar and was still throbbing with the effort.

A similar sight greeted me, unexpectedly, at the opposite end of the bed. The baby's rosy head was visible, and I watched in fixated fascination as its shoulders and then its whole body plopped out onto the bed. It was a boy! His body was smeared with white, waxy vernix and he was plump and perfect, his little arms and legs unfolding and wriggling with life. Mrs Hollingworth let out a noise that was a cross between a whoop and a wail as her baby was delivered, and I stood transfixed as the midwife set about cutting the scarlet-faced baby's cord while telling Mrs Hollingworth she'd done the most tremendous job *ever*, and was the mother of a lovely new son.

She had indeed done a marvellous job, I thought. I became aware that I was standing there holding my breath with my mouth open, gaping at the scene that had unfolded before me. I was utterly astonished that the female body could stretch to such proportions, to deliver such a bouncing baby into the world so seamlessly.

The little boy let out a lusty cry, and I wanted to cry myself. I was shaking a little, and felt a powerful surge of excitement course through my body. It was a feeling I recognised but couldn't quite place. Later, I realised the last time I had been flooded with so much adrenaline was when I was watching The Beatles perform in concert at the Apollo in Ardwick, Manchester, in 1965. It was absolutely electrifying, and I screamed and screamed as if my life depended it on it, just like all the other girls.

Now I felt just as invigorated and ecstatic. Childbirth is the most incredible phenomenon, and in that moment, in that delivery room, my ambition was truly ignited.

'I think I'd like to be a midwife,' I said breathlessly to Graham that night on the phone. 'It was just fantastic to see a new life, a new little person being born.'

Saying the word 'midwife' out loud seemed to validate my decision. Until now, I hadn't been sure where my nursing training would lead me. After all, I had wanted to quit just a couple of months earlier, and when I stood in Miss Bell's office with my resignation letter it had felt like exactly the right thing to do. Working at St Mary's had made me feel much better about my career and my future, and now I could see that becoming a midwife was *the* job for me. It was exactly what I should do and, more importantly, it was exactly what I wanted to do. The certainty in my mind thrilled me, and I felt the happiest I had in a long time.

'That sounds wonderful,' Graham said when he got a word in edgeways. 'I knew you'd find your niche, my little nurse. But how do you go about becoming a midwife?'

There was a hint of worry in his voice, as Graham knew full well that my placement at St Mary's was coming to an end soon. I had more than a year of my nurse's training to complete and four tough exams to pass before I would become a qualified State Registered Nurse, or SRN, in September 1969. I would also have to complete a further three months' work at the MRI after qualifying to become an official MRI nurse, as that was the rule. All told, that would take me to December 1969, and it was still only June 1968.

'I'm not sure,' I said. 'I'll just have to grit my teeth and get through the rest of my placements as best I can. I'll have to keep telling myself it won't be forever. I'm going to see about working at St Mary's after I qualify. I'm going to find out what you have to do to train as a midwife.'

A few weeks later I found myself walking the familiar path to Miss Bell's office. She had asked me to report to her immediately after finishing my placement at St Mary's. I'd left the maternity hospital with a heavy heart, wishing I could stay and learn, and dreading my return to the MRI.

'Come in, Nurse Lawton, and do take a seat,' Miss Bell said when she answered my timid knock on her door.

I walked in nervously and sat down, watching Miss Bell reach purposefully into her desk drawer. She pulled out my resignation letter and waved it before me. For a moment fear made my heart contract. What if she had decided to accept my resignation after all?

'What shall I do with this?' she asked.

In that moment I knew there was only one answer she wanted to hear, and I knew wholeheartedly it was the right answer to give.

'Tear it up!' I said, a relieved smile on my face.

'That's right,' Miss Bell said, before ripping the letter cleanly in two and depositing it in the wastepaper bin beneath her desk.

I felt thankful and exhilarated all at once. I would work hard to pass my exams and gain my qualifications, and then I could train to become a midwife.

'Thank you, Miss Bell,' I said politely. 'I feel much happier now.'

At the time I saw it as a nuisance that I had many more placements to fulfil before I could pursue my training as a midwife. I viewed my final year as a means to an end, not realising how much more invaluable experience I was going to amass along the way.

Within days, I was dismayed to find myself heading back to Booth Hall Children's Hospital to work in the dreaded burns unit, no less. I gritted my teeth and vowed to do my best, although I could not have asked for a worse placement and prayed I would not faint in front of the children again.

'Welcome, Nurse Lawton,' Sister Pattinson said, laying a gentle hand on my shoulder, when I arrived for my first shift. She was a trim, tall lady who spoke in a sweet voice. I wasn't used to a sister being so tactile but I liked it, and thankfully she helped put me at my ease straight away.

This was to be a ten-week placement, and I had been allocated a room in the nurses' home at nearby Monsall Hospital in Newton Heath, North Manchester, as it was close to Booth Hall. Founded in 1871, the grand old Monsall was an isolation hospital that specialised in the care of patients with tuberculosis and infectious diseases.

The idea of leaving my familiar digs at the MRI and living in the grounds of such a place hardly appealed, and I begged Graham to come and visit at least twice a week.

'I don't know about the patients,' I grumbled, 'I think it's me who's being put in isolation.'

'I'll visit as often as I can,' Graham said. 'Will I be able to see your room this time?'

I laughed. 'Don't be daft.' Men were never permitted inside any nurses' home, ever. 'But I'm told there is a communal sitting room where we can welcome visitors.'

'That's fine,' Graham said. 'As long as we can see each other.'

I knew he meant it. Although we had been dating for almost four years we had still never slept together. Graham was a true gent and had never put me under any pressure to do so. We giggled when we sometimes saw other nurses emerging, breathless, from their boyfriends' Minis and Capris in the most dimly lit corners of the MRI car park, but we could only guess at what they got up to. Graham and I had an unspoken understanding that we would wait until we got married before having sex. Until then I felt flattered and comfortable in the knowledge he would willingly drive all the way across Manchester just to come and hold my hand and give me a cuddle and a goodnight kiss.

I was very pleasantly surprised when I was shown to my new accommodation. The furniture was dark and old but my bedroom was on the ground floor and had patio windows that filled the room with light and gave me a lovely view over the most beautiful gardens. Pink roses nodded colourfully between lush evergreens and the sun glinted through the trees, projecting what looked like a pretty dappled rug over the grass. It was such a peaceful and idyllic scene that it helped me imagine I might perhaps enjoy my time here after all.

A taxi took me to Booth Hall each day and I was to wear my own uniform, which was disappointing as the staff nurses had pretty gingham uniforms that I was quite envious of. Not only that, I soon realised they were allowed to swap their white aprons for red, yellow and blue ones when they served food to the children. I thought it was a lovely touch, though it surprised me as it seemed so frivolous compared to the strict and bland uniform regulations I was used to at the MRI.

'I have three special patients I would like you to meet,' Sister Pattinson told me on my first full day, steering me gently from her office.

I prepared myself for the unbearable mixture of stifling heat and the overwhelming stench of livid flesh and clammy Vaseline that had become my abiding memory of the burns unit, but again I found myself surprised. The stuffy temperature and sickly smell could not have been described as pleasant by any means, but the ward wasn't half as bad as I remembered it from my previous, truncated visit.

As I was taken on a little tour I felt my shoulders relax slightly, and I allowed myself to inhale fully through my nostrils, smiling with relief when the ward air hit my lungs without causing my head or my stomach to react.

'This is Karen,' Sister Pattinson said, slipping through a yellow curtain decorated with swirls of blue and orange snakes. 'Karen, this is Nurse Lawton.'

Karen didn't turn to look at me, for which I was grateful, as I needed a moment to compose myself. The little girl, who was no more than five years old, was lying face down on a bed that appeared to have been specially made for her from Plaster of Paris, as it was moulded perfectly beneath her little body. The entire back of Karen's body, from her head to her heels, was covered in dressings and bandages. I registered with some shock that her hands were bound, too, and she was strapped to her bespoke bed by a pair of cloth belts, rendering her immobile. Karen was sucking a drink of orange squash through a straw, held for her by a nurse who sat on a stool by the little girl's head. In between sucks, Karen writhed and sobbed.

Sister Pattinson tilted her head towards me and whispered softly that Karen had fallen backwards into a shallow bath of scalding hot water. Her mother had slipped out of the bathroom for a matter of seconds before returning to switch on the cold tap, but it was too late. Karen was so badly burned that she needed a series of complicated and painful skin grafts to the back of her head, trunk and thighs, and would be in here for many months.

'One of your duties will be to help feed Karen, to read to her and generally try to help make her as comfortable as possible,' she said. 'Do you think you can do that?'

'Yes,' I said, looking at the matted mess of hair and flesh and gauze on the back of Karen's head. I wanted to help her in any way I could. I crouched so I could see Karen's pretty face. She looked withdrawn, but when I said 'hello' she mouthed 'hello' back to me.

The next patient I met was Michael, a little African boy who was three years old and had tightly sprung, jet-black curls and eyes like a couple of Maltesers. He was adorable, and I was very upset to hear that he had been burnt after pulling a pan of hot milk from the stove. He had bandages covering the whole of the left side of his face and eye, but Sister Pattinson assured me that he had been extremely fortunate and his injuries were not too severe.

'Michael likes to play with the farm set and Tonka Trucks,' Sister said affectionately. 'Sometimes distraction is the best medicine for the little ones. I'm sure you'll be very good at that.'

Finally, I was introduced to Gillian. She was four years old and was described by Sister Pattinson as a Mongol, which back then was the common term used to describe someone with Down's Syndrome. Gillian had been born to an 'elderly prima gravida' – an older first-time mother – who was apparently not coping well with having a child so very late in life.

After my shift I looked up 'elderly prima gravida' in one of my books and discovered the term was given to a first-time mother over the age of thirty-five, which to my young mind did seem extremely old to be having your first baby. I'd never come across a mother who had had a child so late in life before, and I imaged poor Gillian's mother to be tired and grey.

'She was trying to help her daughter when the accident happened, and is devastated,' Sister Pattinson explained. 'Gillian was constipated so her mother decided to warm her potty in an effort to help her empty her bowels. Unfortunately, the metal pot was heated to such a high temperature that it burnt a nasty ring round Gillian's bottom.'

Gillian flashed me a smile that belied the pain she must have been feeling beneath the intricate patchwork of dressings swathed around her. In her hand she had a battered old Rupert Bear annual, with Rupert playing in the snow on the front cover. She thrust it towards me expectantly, and bellowed 'Hello Nurse!' very loudly.

Sister Pattinson gave me a little nod of approval. 'You can start here, Nurse Lawton,' she smiled. 'But be warned, that book is well loved and Gillian will have you reading it from cover to cover ten times over if you let her!'

I phoned my mum later that evening, as I had promised to let her know how I was settling in at Booth Hall. I told her I was enjoying the experience much more than I'd imagined I would.

'Your father and I have always thought you would be very good with little ones, being such a caring girl,' Mum told me. 'I know he doesn't say a lot, but your dad is very proud of you, you know. We both are. You're a credit to us, Linda.'

'Thanks, Mum,' I said, feeling tears well in my eyes. 'I feel very lucky. When you see what some of these poor children are going through, it breaks your heart and makes you realise that you don't have any problems at all by comparison, not really.'

I soon became adept at changing dressings on the burns unit. It wasn't such a hard job once I got used to it, and the children rewarded me in spades with their little smiles, or by unexpectedly placing their hand in mine.

I spent a great deal of time reading to both Karen and Gillian. Karen cried a lot, and it broke my heart that I couldn't tend to her auburn hair, which remained matted and tangled for the entirety of my placement, but her scalp was so badly burned it was impossible to wash or even gently brush her hair.

Gillian was eventually allowed to go home after six weeks of treatment to her burnt bottom, and the day before she was due to be discharged I plucked up the courage to confide in Sister Pattinson that I was a little concerned about her on-going welfare.

I had met Gillian's mother several times by now, and had seen that her age was not the issue at all. Even though she was probably about forty, she was hardly the wrinkled old woman I'd imagined an 'elderly prima gravida' might be. However, she was painfully shy to the point of being awkward, and seemed to have a great deal of trouble communicating with Gillian, let alone coping with her.

'Don't worry yourself, Linda,' Sister Pattinson said, rubbing the tops of my arms in a motherly way. 'They say every cloud has a silver lining, and in actual fact I believe it has been some-thing of a blessing that Gillian has come to our attention. It seems neither of her parents have been coping very well with her and her mother in particular is a slow learner, but now they are going to receive help at home.'

'Oh, that's really good,' I said, feeling pleased my instincts had been accurate.

Of the three of them, it was little Michael who really left his mark on me – but not in a way I'd anticipated. One evening he climbed out of his cot and walked towards me, crying, with his arms outstretched.

'Whatever's the matter, Michael?' I asked, scooping him onto my hip in the dimly lit ward. He was dressed in nothing but a terry nappy, which was normal as the ward was kept so warm.

'I've got doo-doo on my leg,' he said shyly, at which point I smelled exactly what he was talking about. Looking down, I saw that my white apron was now streaked with brown, and both Michael I and needed to go post-haste to the bathroom.

'So-wry, Nurse,' he said, hiding his face in my sleeve.

'It doesn't matter at all,' I said, which was the truth. I had dealt with worse, and I had clean hands and a fresh apron on in no time. The burns unit had been an experience, and one I did not regret after all.

Chapter Seven

*'Unless you ladder your stockings, to my mind you haven't
made a good job of dealing with a cardiac arrest!'*

My next two placements were to be on a cardiac ward, and
then in the Casualty department. It was the autumn of 1968
and I was a third year now, which meant I was allowed to
wear three white stripes of bias binding on my sleeve. This
provided a boost to my growing confidence as well as to my
bank balance, as my pay rose automatically from £27 to £31 a
month after my accommodation was paid for.

On my first day on the cardiac ward, I was told to report to
Sister Hyde, who I'd heard from Linda and Anne was a 'right
character'.

'Oh, there you are, Nurse Lawton,' a deep voice bellowed
from a side room as I entered the ward.

I followed the low boom curiously and to my astonishment
I discovered Sister Hyde lying prostrate on the floor, chunky
legs protruding like logs from beneath her skirt. Once again, I
found myself standing and staring, mouth wide open, but this
time it was in utter surprise rather than fascination.

'Come in, come in. Don't just stand there!' Sister Hyde
beckoned, before laying her head back down and starting to
thrash her thick arms and jerk her large chest about.

I realised, to my amusement, that she was pretending to
have a heart attack, the purpose of which was to instruct a

group of first- and second-year students in resuscitation techniques.

'Put your hand on my chest,' she was saying to a timid-looking second year. 'Don't be afraid to give it a right big push. Get stuck in, girl, go on!'

Addressing her wide-eyed audience, Sister Hyde shouted dramatically: 'Unless you ladder your stockings, to my mind you haven't made a good job of dealing with a cardiac arrest!'

I warmed instantly to Sister Hyde. She certainly was a real character, and over the next few weeks I loved working with her. I learned that she smoked incessantly in the kitchen off the side of the ward, asking us students to give her the nod if Matron was in the vicinity. Unlike the majority of the other sisters, who were spinsters, Sister Hyde had a husband and a busy life outside the hospital. We all liked her and she would often make us young nurses sandwiches, or 'butties' as she called them, so as to keep up our strength up on the ward.

'You won't have the strength to ladder your stockings, let alone jolt a heart into action, if you don't put fuel in your belly,' was one of her favourite mantras.

'Get this butty inside you and then go on and get it sorted out,' she said to me regularly, thrusting a brown bread sandwich made with Marmite or meat paste in my direction. Bed-making and taking temperatures often had to wait while I did as I was told and wolfed down my butty.

My confidence grew still further under Sister Hyde's strong wing, and I found myself holding my head a little bit higher each day. I still would have much preferred to be looking after new mothers and their babies at St Mary's, but compared to some of my experiences at the MRI, being on the cardiac ward was not bad at all.

The patients proved a boon to my self-esteem. The way the men flirted outrageously with the young nurses in films like *Carry on Nurse* was certainly not a true reflection of what went on in real life. Almost without exception, male patients of all ages viewed us nurses like angels and treated us with the utmost respect. They thanked us profusely for every perceived kindness, whether we were giving injections, gathering bedpans or simply handing out mugs of Ovaltine at bedtime.

I began to really enjoy night shifts. As a first and second year I'd found them a bit scary. The night sister was usually in her office during the shift and there were scarcely any qualified nurses on the ward. I'd often felt out of my depth and vulnerable with just the older students keeping an eye on me, and I'd worn myself out with worry as much as with the work. As a third year, however, I'd sit at the table under the green light and feel competent and capable as I tallied the fluid input and output charts, helped younger students with their queries, wrote up reports or prepared drugs for the patients.

One night, when the ward was in perfect order and all the patients were sleeping, I was congratulating myself on my efforts when a new arrival was wheeled in by an apologetic porter. The large, middle-aged man had survived a suspected heart attack, but he was reeking of whisky and nothing could be done until he'd sobered up. He was lifted into a bed and I hoped he would just sleep it off, but before long the patient began to stir.

'Where's the toilet, Nurse?' he shouted as he threw off his bedclothes and began swaggering along the ward, waking half the other patients in the process.

'I can get you a bottle if you like,' I said, rushing over, but he brushed me aside and lurched towards the bathroom. I followed him, concerned he might fall and injure himself, but to my surprise he swung round clumsily without warning, grabbed me by my collar and slammed me against a door.

'Oi! Pack it in!' a male voice ordered.

'Watch it, mate!' another warned.

'Don't lay a finger on her!' a third pitched in.

Almost before I could register the pain shooting across my shoulderblades, all three of these male patients had leapt to my aid, and my pyjama-clad protectors bundled the protesting drunk back into bed while I slipped away to alert Sister. I was shaken up but thanks to my chivalrous patients I escaped with nothing more than a ruffled collar, a sore back and a little bruised pride. The next day one of the male patients handed me a box of Milk Tray.

'My wife brought these in for you,' he said. 'She said I was to give them to "that lovely little nurse".'

A few days afterwards I told Graham what had happened and he was naturally concerned.

'It's not right that you're put in danger like that,' he said. 'Anything could have happened!'

'Don't worry, it's very unusual,' I replied, truthfully. 'The patients are generally absolutely lovely. They treat us like little princesses, honestly. Some of the men even offer to help dish out the cups of tea at 4 p.m., because they can see how hard we work and they want to help us.'

This conversation reminded me of an incident soon after I started my second year and was doing a night shift on a female medical ward.

'Remember Mrs Thurlow?' I asked Graham, wanting to ease his concern. 'Now *she's* a typical patient, not this clumsy drunken man.'

I reminded Graham of the story, though I was sure he'd heard it before. It happened after I had distributed two sleeping pills to a middle-aged lady called Mrs Thurlow in bed seven, who had nipped to the toilet while I made my round.

Everyone slept soundly on the ward that night, and before I finished my shift the next morning I filled in my report and remarked that it had been a 'peaceful night, without incident'. However, flicking through the Kardex file I spotted, to my horror, that alongside Mrs Thurlow's name in bold red letters was a warning: 'DO NOT GIVE SEDATION'.

'My heart jumped into my throat and I ran to bed seven as quickly as my legs would carry me,' I told Graham, laughing now at the memory. I had been mightily relieved to see Mrs Thurlow propped up comfortably with her eyes open, squinting at a crossword.

'Mrs Thurlow!' I began. 'Did you ... are you ...'

'Are you on about the sleeping pills?' she chuckled.

'Yes!' I stuttered.

To my utter relief, Mrs Thurlow leaned towards me conspiratorially and whispered behind her hand, 'Don't worry, pet. I never took 'em. I threw 'em down the toilet. Knew I weren't meant to.' She gave me a wink and turned her gaze back to her crossword.

Those were the typical patients, I assured Graham when I'd finished reliving the story. Typical patients were kind and genuinely appreciative of the care they were receiving. I hoped I'd meet many more like Mrs Thurlow during my time in Casualty, which was where I was off to on my next placement.

* * *

I could see immediately that working in Casualty was going to be more like running a conveyor belt than working on a ward, and from the start I missed the rapport I had come to enjoy with the patients. Each hour brought a relentless blare of emergency sirens, breathless paramedics, staggering drunks and victims of all manner of accidents, some unlikely in the extreme.

'My daft husband's got his sleeve rings caught in 'is hair, Nurse,' one agitated woman explained on my very first shift. 'Don't know what he was playing at; fooling around, no doubt.'

I looked at her husband curiously. Embedded in his thick mop of wavy hair was one of those metal garter rings used by men to tuck their shirt sleeves up their arms, to keep their cuffs from becoming soiled while working. I've no idea how he managed it; it was practically knitted to his head.

'He works at the printing press in Oldham,' she said quite desperately. 'He's meant to clock on in 'alf an hour.'

'Let's get a pair of scissors, then,' I said.

I was too busy to question why they had taken the trouble to come into Casualty. They clearly wanted to salvage either the haircut or the sleeve ring or both, though neither looked particularly precious. I deduced that one of them had to go, and decided it was easier to sacrifice the hair, which looked in need of a cut anyhow. The wife looked close to tears as I cropped the thick silver ring out of her husband's hair, leaving him with an unattractive bald patch above his left ear.

I handed her the thatched ring without further ado and packed the couple on their way, thankful I could now attend to patients in real need of medical attention.

'Perhaps you should have gone to a barber shop instead,' I wanted to shout after them, but I held my tongue and thought,

'If only Miss Morgan or Sister Bridie were here, they'd have given them what for!'

The following week I'd just started my shift at 9 p.m. on a Saturday night when I heard the wail of an ambulance siren and the sound of screeching tyres outside. A small girl called Tabitha was stretchered in, followed by two hysterical women, who identified themselves as the girl's mother and aunt.

'Nurse Lawton will take care of you,' I heard the male charge nurse, Dennis, tell them as he herded us together. 'Follow her over there, into the side room.'

I had never come across a male nurse before. I could instantly see how a man like him, who clearly stood for no messing, could be extremely useful in Casualty, but on this occasion I found his manner unnecessarily rude.

As I gently ushered the wailing women into a side room and fetched them cups of tea, I felt an overwhelming urge to make them feel better.

'There, there,' I soothed. 'Tabitha will be all right.'

The girl's distraught mother wiped her eyes with the backs of her trembling hands and looked me straight in the eye. 'I do 'ope you're right, Nurse,' she said. 'I do 'ope so.'

As she spoke I sensed some tension falling away, but the poor woman's ruddy face was still etched with worry.

Several hours later I heard the most dreadful news: Tabitha had bled to death. She was just five years old and had been hit by a car, and the injuries she sustained were too catastrophic for her to survive.

I never saw Tabitha's mother again, at least not in person, but every night for weeks and weeks afterwards I saw her devastated face in my dreams. I saw the little glint of hope I gave that mother with my careless words. False hope. I had no idea how bad Tabitha's injuries were and I gave her mother false hope with my erroneous comfort. How wrong had I been? I vowed never, ever to make that mistake again.

One evening before bed I felt the need to 'confess' to someone what I'd done. I'd not told Graham about Tabitha, which was unusual, but after almost three years of comforting me though my training I felt I was putting a little too much on him. I didn't want him to think I wasn't coping this far down the line.

It was 1969 now, and we were getting married later in the year. We'd set the date for 22 November, two months after I would hopefully have qualified as an SRN, and during the period when I would be completing my final three months' work at the MRI.

I decided to have a chat to Linda about what had happened with Tabitha. She might help me cope with it. I tapped on her door and she opened it slowly, ashen-faced.

'Whatever's the matter?' I asked. She threw her arms around my neck and began to cry.

'I'm so sorry,' she said. 'Really, I'm so sorry to make such a fuss.'

I let Linda take her time. She told me, in a series of sobs, that her mum had lost her long battle with cancer and the family had decided to move back to Scotland. Linda's long-term boyfriend had secured a job in Edinburgh and she was planning to complete her training in a Scottish hospital, after taking a period of compassionate leave.

I felt desperately sorry for Linda. She had helped nurse her mother for years, never once complaining about their circumstances. I found it hard enough coping with the deaths of patients on the wards, and I couldn't begin to comprehend what she was going through. Just the thought of losing some-one so close made me shiver. It was devastating and I wished I could do something to help ease Linda's pain.

At the same time I was upset about Linda leaving the MRI. I knew I would miss her tremendously. Out of all the student nurses, she had become my closest friend. She always had a tale to tell and a knack of lifting my spirits. Linda had also earned a reputation for sticking up for herself against some of the more tyrannical sisters, which I admired and respected. I was losing a good friend and ally, and I felt the loss acutely.

I also felt a strong pang of nostalgia. Linda's departure would signal the end of an era, the end of our time together as student nurses. Although I had spent hours on the phone tell-ing Graham how much I couldn't wait to finish at the MRI and move out of the nurses' home, I realised I would miss being a student. That reaction surprised me. I'd got used to my life, I suppose, and for the most part I was enjoying being a senior amongst the student nurses.

There was an element of fear in my response to Linda's news, too. We were all moving on, one way or another. The future was uncertain, and through Linda's tear-filled eyes I could see that life never stood still, and that at times it could be very tough indeed.

The last six months of my training were arduous as I studied hard for my final exams and completed two more placements. The first was in theatre, where I was put under the wing of Sister Helen Wood. I had met her before, many months earlier, when I was asked to provide an extra pair of hands during a haemorrhoid operation. Then, I'd been bowled over by her to the point where it was fair to say I idolised her. She was not only extremely good at her job, she was absolutely beautiful too, with eyes like lamps that bathed you in a warm, inspiring glow.

I had helped Sister Wood sterilise and prepare the instruments for the operation and hung on her every word as she taught me how to 'scrub' by washing up to my elbows, and to put on the theatre gown, apron, mask, hat and gloves in the correct order. Inside the theatre I watched in admiration as she passed the skilful surgeon, Mr Thornton, exactly the right implement at precisely the right moment. It was clear Mr Thornton held Sister Wood in high regard too, as he grumbled to her afterwards, 'Why can't they all be like you?'

Mr Thornton was an extremely well-respected surgeon and it was common knowledge that he did not suffer fools. I had felt honoured to be asked to scrub for him on that first occasion. In fact, I was so taken with the experience I barely focused on the operation in hand – although to tell the truth I wasn't particularly enamoured with seeing what became of the bunch of grape-like haemorrhoids he removed from the poor patient. My main responsibility was to count the number of swabs in and out before and after the operation, lest one be left inside.

I remember Nessa asking me, wide-eyed, what it had been like to witness an actual real-life operation, and having to confess that I was so enthralled by Sister Wood's flawless performance and the ceremony of the theatre with the bright lights, curtains and white gloves that I barely focused on Mr Thornton's surgical skills.

As I was now a third year, Sister Wood explained that this time I would be working as the senior nurse in theatre, and as such it would be my responsibility to pass Mr Thornton the correct instruments as and when he called for them. The operation was a mastectomy on a patient with breast cancer, which Sister Wood talked me through in some detail.

'Do you think you can manage that?' she asked.

I was nervous, but I also felt very privileged to have been given this opportunity. I gave an enthusiastic smile and an emphatic 'yes', ignoring the little voice inside me that wanted to say: 'Help! What if I make a mistake?'

Since I had watched Sister Wood in action, I knew that Mr Thornton appreciated nurses who had the correct instrument to hand almost before he called for it, a standard I knew I could not deliver as I had never worked alone with him before, and had no experience of what a mastectomy required.

I was anxious, and I could feel my pulse throbbing against the strings of my mask as I finished scrubbing up. Mr Thornton was an enormous man, with bright red hair and a thick, severely clipped moustache. Beneath his gown he had a barrel of a stomach and, if you dared glance at the incongruous twinkle in his blue eyes, I swear you could see the spark of a furious fire. I'd heard countless tales of Mr Thornton bawling at nurses and, though I had never witnessed an explosion myself, I couldn't help imagining him as a giant grenade, his red hair and flashing eyes already ignited. As I stepped into his theatre, scrubbed and willing to serve, ready or not, I felt sure he was about to blow.

Mr Thornton barely acknowledged me as he huffed and puffed his way through the long operation. I delivered each and every instrument he required as swiftly as humanly possible, but he was clearly not pleased. He was used to the immaculate Sister Wood, with her near-psychic ability to pre-empt his every request, and he let it be known I was not up to scratch. Tut-tutting and sighing, he snatched knives and swabs from me with astonishing rudeness, and I could feel my nerves stretching taut like elastic. My cheeks were burning and my hands were shaking but I bit my lip and told myself to concentrate on giving him the instruments he asked for, or the situation would get a whole lot worse.

'Promise me, Linda, you will always work hard for your living.' I heard Sister Mary Francis's voice in my ear, and my own response that I most certainly would. I was working very hard here, so why did Mr Thornton have to make it so difficult for me to succeed? Surely he had been brought up to believe good manners were as important as hard work, just as I had?

'Receiver!' Mr Thornton growled. I reached for a small bowl and then changed my mind, catastrophically. It must have taken me less than a second to pick up the larger bowl on the other side of the tray, but I was too late.

'Take this!' Mr Thornton hissed. I felt it before I saw it: a warm, soft, bloody lump hit me right in the heart. I watched, horrified, as it slid down my apron and slapped on the theatre floor at my feet. It was a severed breast. Mr Thornton had thrust it at me so impatiently he had missed the bowl completely and hit me instead. He had actually thrown the cancerous breast at me!

I burst into tears and ran out of the theatre as fast as I could, pulling off my blood-streaked apron as if it were contaminated. I knew I shouldn't have done this, but I also knew there was another theatre nurse in there who could take over, so I didn't stop myself.

I was as disgusted and embarrassed as I was upset, and I couldn't help sobbing noisily. After the operation was finished Sister Wood's arm appeared around my shoulder, and I blubbed like a baby in her arms.

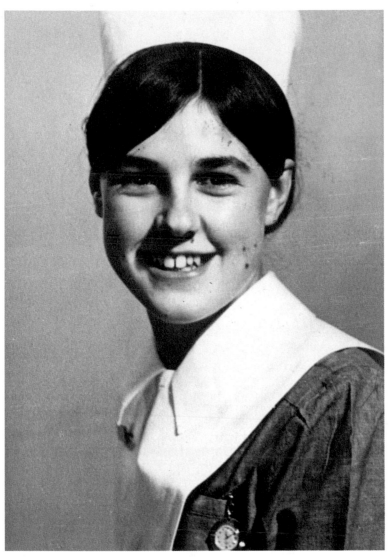

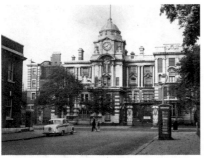

Above: This was taken during my first year of training at the Manchester Royal Infirmary (*left*), aged 18. I can't help but chuckle at how young and inexperienced I was! Despite nursing not being for me, I'm so grateful for all the invaluable experience and knowledge I gained there, and for the many amazing people I met along the way.

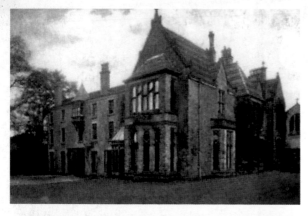

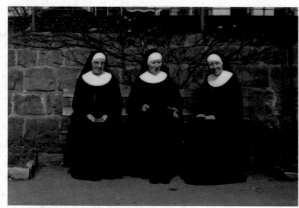

Top: Harrytown High School in Romiley, Cheshire, where my dream of becoming a nurse began.

Left: 'Please promise me, Linda, that you will always work hard.' The words of Sister Mary Francis (far left) still echo clearly in my mind. I hope I've made her proud.

Below: Sixth form at Harrytown. I'm kneeling in the front row, fourth from the left.

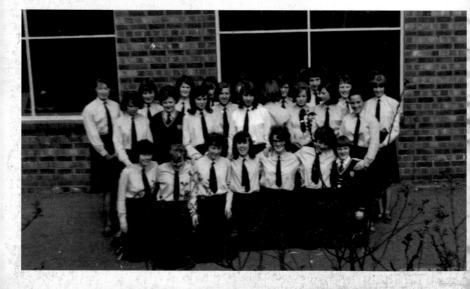

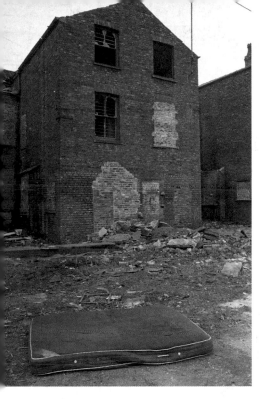

I soon learned that life wasn't all rosy. Some parts of Manchester were terribly poor, and these streets are typical of the ones I'd race down on my Honda to the aid of women like Moira Petty, whose story still haunts me today.

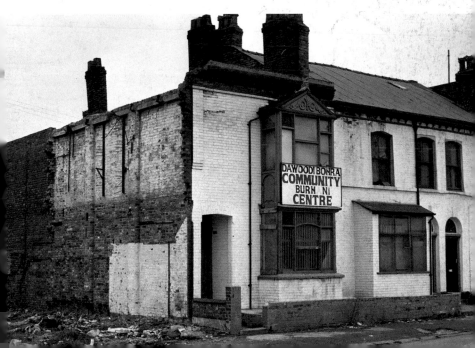

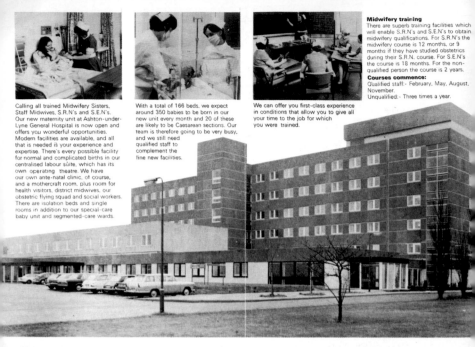

Calling all trained Midwifery Sisters, Staff Midwives, S.R.N's and S.E.N's. Our new maternity unit at Ashton-under-Lyne General Hospital is now open and offers you wonderful opportunities. Modern facilities are available, and all that is needed is your experience and expertise. There's every possible facility for normal and complicated births in our centralised labour suite, which has its own operating theatre. We have our own ante-natal clinic, of course, and a mothercraft room, plus room for health visitors, district midwives, our obstetric flying squad and social workers. There are isolation beds and single rooms in addition to our special-care baby unit and segmented-care wards.

With a total of 166 beds, we expect around 350 babies to be born in our new unit every month and 20 of these are likely to be Caesarean sections. Our team is therefore going to be very busy, and we still need qualified staff to complement the fine new facilities.

We can offer you first-class experience in conditions that allow you to give all your time to the job for which you were trained.

Midwifery training
There are superb training facilities which will enable S.R.N's and S.E.N's to obtain midwifery qualifications. For S.R.N's the midwifery course is 12 months, or 9 months if they have studied obstetrics during their S.R.N. course. For S.E.N's the course is 18 months. For the non-qualified person the course is 2 years.
Courses commence:
Qualified staff:- February, May, August, November.
Unqualified:- Three times a year.

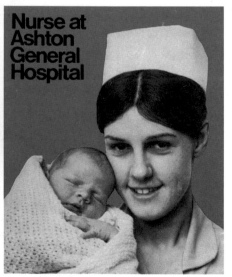

Nurse at Ashton General Hospital

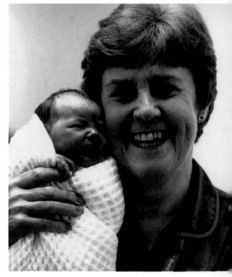

Top and above left: A copy of the brochure with my photo used to advertise the new maternity unit at Ashton General Hospital, later renamed Tameside Hospital, where I still work today (*above right*). I was so proud to have been chosen to represent the hospital; it was a real stamp of approval after all the hard years of training. It's such a privilege to be a midwife, which is why – forty years later – I continue to do the job I love.

'It was grotesque,' I gasped. 'I can't believe that just happened. That poor lady, too. How could he do such a thing to her, to me, to anybody?'

Moments later Mr Thornton crashed out of the theatre. He looked for all the world like a crazed villain stepping out of a horror film. He was splattered with blood, large globules of sweat were pricking his forehead and his eyes were ablaze.

'What's she crying for?' he barked. 'I wouldn't waste my breath shouting if I didn't think she had potential!'

It took me quite a while to digest what he had said, and to accept and understand that he had paid me something of a compliment, albeit a very cruelly delivered one. I went on to scrub for Mr Thornton several more times, and though he never treated me with the reverence he clearly reserved for Sister Wood, there was an understanding between us after that. I was at least worthy of scrubbing for him, which was a huge vote of confidence from such a demanding surgeon.

On the Saturday night before Linda left for Scotland in the spring of 1969, Jo, Anne, Nessa and I took her out to the Twisted Wheel in Whitworth Street. We'd all been there before and agreed it was the best dance club in town, though we'd never managed to go as a group before.

'Isn't it funny?' Anne said wistfully. 'When you look back to when we first met, thrown together in our little group, I imagined we'd be out together all the time.'

'How naïve we were!' Jo chortled. 'Who'd have thought we'd have to work so hard? I think I've spent more Saturday evenings either doing nights or catching up on sleep and study than I have going out dancing.'

Nessa nodded in agreement, though we all knew she was happier with her nose in a book than she was dancing. Despite their different personalities, she, Jo and Anne had decided to move into a flat together at the end of their training, as they all hoped to secure jobs at the MRI. They'd invited me to join them, but nobody had been surprised when I told them Graham and I had set a date for our wedding and intended to live near our parents' in Stalybridge after our marriage.

'Haven't we had some laughs though, eh?' Linda said cheerfully.

She wanted to go out on a high, and we all did our best to give her a good send off. We'd certainly dressed for the occasion. Everybody was wearing a mini dress and brightly coloured tights. Anne had teased her hair into a beehive and even Nessa had spent an hour getting ready, pencilling neat black flicks at the corners of her eyes and painting her lips sugar-pink.

I was wearing a tight-fitting burnt-orange leather jacket I'd fallen in love with in Lewis's department store. It had a military collar with press-studs and two little zip-up pockets on the front. It had cost me the extortionate sum of £21 – practically a month's salary.

'Are you not going to take your coat off, Linda?' the girls teased, knowing it was my pride and joy and I wouldn't be parted from it for the world.

'Honestly, Linda, you're so extravagant,' they mocked, knowing how frugally we had all lived for almost three years and that I was certainly not in the habit of splashing out.

'What would our superiors say about my frivolity?' I joked, provoking a string of mickey-takes from all but Nessa.

'You reckless, foolish girl!' Jo declared, putting on old Miss Morgan's stern clipped tone of voice.

'May the Lord have mercy on you!' Anne exaggerated in Sister Bridie's Irish brogue.

'Fetch me the scissors – I can't give CPR through a jacket like that!' Linda laughed, taking off Sister Hyde to a tee.

'We've certainly had some fun,' Jo said, suddenly cracking up as she remembered one of her favourite tales. 'I don't think I'll ever laugh as much as I did that time when Anne and I mixed up all the dentures on M5.'

Anne, chubby as ever, almost rolled off her stool she began to chuckle so hard. 'Me neither,' she hooted. 'I think it was when I heard you saying, "Mr Norton, would you mind trying this pair for size?" that I completely lost it!' Slapping her thigh, Anne added: 'The worst of it was, this was the same poor man we'd given a cottage pie to, forgetting he was a strict vegetarian. Shame on us! By the time he'd finished and told us it was the best vegetarian pie he'd ever tasted, we didn't have the heart to admit it was nothing of the sort!'

We laughed all night, drinking orange squash and dancing in the basement, where there were lots of iron wheels decorating the painted brick walls. The DJ sat behind a sort of cage and played some of our favourite 78s by The Beatles and The Dave Clark Five, which we had a good bop to. We talked about everything under the sun. Concorde had recently made its maiden flight, which was on everyone's lips, and we fantasised about where we would fly to if ever we won the Pools and could afford supersonic travel.

'I would follow The Beatles on their next world tour,' I said firmly. 'Vidal Sassoon would do my hair while I lounged back and watched *The Graduate* on a giant screen!'

The other girls made up similarly alluring scenarios. Jean Shrimpton and Mary Quant would come aboard to give fashion advice *en route* to 'Flower Power' concerts in America (though none of us really knew what happened at such events, beside the fact they always looked very hip and happening on news reports). Nessa, always the more intellectual of the group, would fly over the Berlin Wall so she could see both East and West Germany at a glance before dropping in on Andy Warhol and Indira Gandhi, to talk about Pop Art and women's rights respectively.

It was fun to dream about being part of the jet-set, but in reality I don't think any of us experienced anything like the full force of the 'Swinging Sixties' in our little corner of Manchester. I certainly didn't. I'd see headlines from time to time about hippies and free love and psychedelic drugs, but those kinds of things seemed a million miles away from the sober, daily grind of my life at the MRI.

I knew I had more freedom and opportunities than my mother had done as a teenager in the Thirties and Forties. I could sense that change was happening more quickly than it used to, and I felt empowered by the women's libbers who were fighting so hard for female equality, especially in the workplace. Their efforts filled me with optimism about my future, but I can't pretend I felt part of a revolution. I was just living my life.

We finished the evening by doing the Twist, joking as we did so that we were probably pretty good at it because we were always on our toes at work, and often contorted into silly positions doing bed baths and bedpans!

'Keep in touch, won't you?' we all said to Linda as we made our way home.

'Course I will!' she said. 'You're not getting rid of me that easily!'

We started to run in our little stiletto heels as we passed the mortuary entrance on the way into the nurses' home. This had become something of a ritual at the end of a night out, because the mortuary workers all looked like Frankenstein's monsters after dark. I enjoyed being out with the girls. We had become very comfortable in each other's company, and that night I felt sure we'd always stay in touch, come what may.

Chapter Eight

'T' Eagle 'as landed'

During my final months as a third year in the summer of 1969 I was back on Sister Craddock's ward for another short placement, which seemed fitting as it had been my very first ward.

As I reported for a night shift with two second-year students, Sister Craddock informed us that most of the patients were in for routine ops and simply needed observation overnight. There was only one exception – a patient with leukaemia called John Fisher. He was in a side ward attached to a chemotherapy drip containing Endoxan, and we'd need to keep an extra eye on him.

'As always, I expect all the charts to tally in the morning, without exception,' she added, shooting each of us a warning glance. 'To make myself plain, that means the amount of water drunk must correlate to the urine output.' Eyeing the second-year students, she handed out a copy of my notes from the previous shift and added: 'I would be very happy if you could take a leaf out of Nurse Lawton's book. Her mathematics is exemplary, and if all my nurses were like her, most of our problems would be solved.'

I felt myself going pink as Sister Craddock went on to deliver her 'cleanliness is next to godliness' lecture for the umpteenth time, but I barely heard her. Her compliment was buzzing round my head, and I could scarcely believe that the second-year students were looking at me in the admiring way I had looked up to the third years such a short time ago.

I floated off on my tea break later that night, leaving a second year in charge of the ward while Sister Craddock retreated to her office, as she often did, with a pile of input and output charts and a sharp pencil.

Nessa was sitting in the canteen sipping warm tea and eating a square of apple pie. 'How are the wedding plans going, Linda?' she asked sweetly. 'It seems so silly, but I've hardly had a chance to ask you.'

'Fine,' I said, realising I didn't have a lot to tell her. 'To tell the truth I've hardly had a chance to think about it myself. I'm going shopping with my mum in a couple of weeks' time to look for a dress and we're having the reception at the Masonic Hall in Ashton. Dad's not a Mason, by the way; we just like the hall. Oh, and Graham and I have found a house!'

Nessa's eyes widened. 'You lucky thing,' she smiled. 'I bet it's lovely. Where is it?'

I explained that the house was an end of terrace in Grey Street, Stalybridge, which we'd bought from Graham's uncle, who owned most of the row and would be living in the house next door. We'd agreed to pay £1,300 for it, with a mortgage of £13 a month. Graham was going to use the cellar to store the vending machines he now bought and sold, having left his car sales job to set up his own company with his brother. We would officially own it three weeks before the wedding, to give us a chance to do it up before we moved in.

'It all sounds so grown-up,' Nessa grinned. 'Good for you, Linda.'

'What about you?' I asked. 'Have you settled on which flat you're having?'

Nessa sighed. 'Er, yes. It's in Didsbury, is riddled with damp and is a complete rip-off, but at least it's a step in the right direction!'

'You'll love it,' I said, meaning it. While I knew I could never have coped without Graham's support, I could see that I'd missed out on the social front a bit, having spent so much time with him. The rest of the girls had grown closer, I sensed. They went out to the university dances together more often, while Graham and I were planning our wedding and our future.

'You're right,' Nessa nodded. 'I'm not too bothered about the state of the flat. I'm just looking forward to the freedom. Three years in a nurses' home is enough for anyone – even a bookworm like me! But you're ever so lucky, Linda. You'll be a married woman and a fully qualified nurse by the end of the year. I'm so pleased for you.'

I drifted back to the ward on a cloud. Nessa was right. I'd come a long way. I remembered my first tentative steps along these corridors, and the way I would pretend I was holding God's hand to help me through the day. Now my hands were free, and I imagined giving myself an imaginary pat on the back. I really should count my lucky stars. If everything went to plan, by the end of the year I would have passed my nursing exams and started training as a midwife at St Mary's. It was too early to approach the maternity hospital at this stage, as I needed to be a qualified nurse before applying for a pupil midwife post, but that day was drawing closer. As each week passed I allowed myself to dream just a little bit more about what it would be like to deliver baby after baby, day in, day out. I couldn't imagine a more rewarding way to earn a living, bringing new life into the world time and time again. I would never tire of that, I was certain.

My day-dreaming came to a crashing halt that night when I returned to the ward to find that John Fisher had passed away suddenly and unexpectedly in my absence. I was absolutely distraught. He had been fine when I left, and I immediately blamed myself for having left a second year in charge while I went on my break.

'I've let a patient die!' I gasped. 'I've killed poor Mr Fisher!' In my shock and panic I imagined I would be dismissed, or even sent to jail! I would never become a midwife, and I would not be able to marry Graham! I began to shake and sob.

Sister Craddock steered me into her office. 'Nurse Lawton, you are an excellent nurse and I will always stand by you, if it is correct to do so. In this instance, there is no blame to be apportioned to anybody. Mr Fisher's death was caused by his cancer, I'm afraid. That is a fact. Do not blame yourself. There is absolutely no need to feel guilty. You went on a perfectly reasonable tea break. Is that perfectly clear?'

I wiped away my tears and nodded uncertainly, feeling relieved but not quite believing her. It was unusual for her to be on night duty, and on reflection I felt very glad someone of her experience had been the night sister on that occasion. I thought I must have a guardian angel looking out for me, and I was comforted by that idea.

Still, it took me weeks to fully accept Sister Craddock's words. Mr Fisher's death played heavily on my heart and I saw his face many, many times in my dreams. Each time I was reminded how fragile and valuable life is and I shuddered at what a heavy burden it was to be a nurse. Midwifery was so much more uplifting, I thought. Dealing with birth instead of death was definitely the way forward for me, and now, more than ever, I couldn't wait to get started.

'Nurse,' hissed Marilyn Barton, 'can I 'ave a word?'

It was 20 July 1969, and for my very last placement I was doing a night shift in charge of a female medical ward.

'Would it be all right if we were to put telly on quietly? I'd like to watch them walking on the moon.'

Hilda Grimsditch in the bed next door pulled her curtain open.

'Couldn't 'elp overhearing, like. I were going t'ask same thing m'self.'

Before I knew it the ward was buzzing.

'It's history in the making,' another lady, Mildred, exclaimed. 'Did you hear that Neil Armstrong earlier? "T" Eagle 'as landed," he said.'

'Put your teeth in, Mildred,' a chortling pensioner with a purple rinse chipped in. ''Ave you 'eard yerself? "T" eagle 'as landed!" I don't suppose the BBC announcer would say it like that!' The ward erupted with laughter.

It was uplifting to have something so positive to watch on the television. The news at that time was often dominated by the Vietnam War, and it always shocked me to see so much devastation, right there on the screen in front of me. It was the first time a war had been televised, and seeing such terrible images was so alien and upsetting, I often tried to avoid the news altogether.

By contrast, the moon landing was a rousing must-see. Excitement had clearly been building since well before my shift started at 9 p.m. As I'd dressed in my uniform I'd tuned in to the

World Service on the little Bush radio in my bedroom, and was thrilled to hear that the Eagle landing craft had touched down on the surface of the Moon at seventeen minutes past eight.

I was as excited as the patients were about seeing the astronauts actually set foot on the moon, which wasn't expected to happen for a good few hours yet.

'I'm sure it can be arranged,' I said. 'You know the night sister doesn't like the television on at all hours, but if we're all in agreement, and all keep quiet, I think we'll be able to watch in the day room.'

A ripple of applause went round the ward and Marilyn, who was the youngest of the patients, agreed to keep her ear tuned to the hospital radio, which was doing its best to keep up with the latest news in amongst the usual hotchpotch of requests and hit parade music.

Just before midnight, Marilyn declared that it was about time we repaired to the nearby day room, where there was a small black-and-white television, donated by a grateful former patient, and a mismatched collection of chairs and faux-leather pouffes.

A few old dears were sound asleep and had not asked to be woken, but the rest of us – about sixteen in total – tiptoed, hobbled and shuffled to the day room in anticipation of this great historic event.

'I feel like a naughty schoolgirl sneakin' off t'ave a midnight feast!' Hilda tittered. 'Who'd a thought I'd be stuck in 'ere 'aving me varicose veins removed when man were landing on the moon? Ya couldn't credit it, could ya?'

I was afraid we might all get into trouble for this, but I couldn't help enjoying the moment and having a little laugh myself. The ladies looked a picture as they settled in front of the television in their colourful collection of flannelette night-ies, quilted bed jackets and fur-lined mules and slippers. Some also wore bandages and dressings and were attached to intra-venous fluids rigged up to stands, but nobody gave two hoots what they looked like. This historic spectacle was all that mattered, and we sat with our eyes glued to the flickering box in the corner of the room.

A couple of patients enjoyed a cigarette and Marilyn gener-ously passed round two paper bags of sweets to share. 'I got my old man to buy these specially for the occasion,' she giggled. 'Guess what we've got?'

'What?' Hilda replied, opening one of the red-and-white striped packets.

'Space Dust and Flying Saucers!' Marilyn chuckled.

Everybody tittered and tucked in – at least those who'd remembered to put their teeth in – and time slipped effort-lessly by.

Some ladies dozed off as I flitted between the day room and the ward, while others refused to take their eyes off the small screen and promised to wake the rest when the big moment finally arrived.

It must have been about 2 a.m. when I heard the familiar tap-tap of the night sister's shoes treading the corridor between the ward and the day room, where I was sitting quietly.

'Matron's coming!' Hilda exclaimed in mock horror, enjoy-ing the drama. I must admit my heart did a little flip, and I was relieved when it was the night sister, and not Miss Bell, who poked her head round the door a few moments later.

'I hope you don't mind ...' I started.

'Not at all,' she replied briskly. 'But let's have no more smoking, ladies. Mrs Spencer and Mrs Clayton, put those cigarettes out quickly, please. Nurse Lawton, if you could fetch the charts and the medication, we can all stay in here.'

I swiftly obliged, while Sister settled herself into an armchair. Moments later we sat transfixed as Neil Armstrong emerged from the Eagle landing craft. We watched, mesmerised, as he set foot on the moon surface and declared dramatically: 'That's one small step for man, one giant leap for mankind.'

The ladies clapped and cheered while sister dutifully shushed them and warned them not to wake the whole hospital. I looked at the fob watch I normally used for the routine task of checking pulse rates. The moon landing was officially recorded at four minutes before 3 a.m. on 21 July, and it was a moment in time I shall never forget.

My own life was leaping forward, too. By now I'd had a discussion with Mr Tate, my tutor, about how I should go about applying to become a pupil midwife. To my surprise, rather than recommending I return to St Mary's, he suggested I might consider applying to Ashton-under-Lyne General Hospital. I would have to pass all my exams first, of course, for which I was studying very hard. I had four to take in total, each lasting three hours, and I was really feeling the pressure.

From a practical point of view, working in Ashton made perfect sense. With Graham now running his vending machine business from home, I did wonder how I would manage to commute into Manchester every day. It would be bad enough using public transport during the daytime, but how would I cope with night shifts? I couldn't expect Graham to give me lifts all the time, as each round trip would take about an hour.

Mr Tate told me that a brand new maternity unit was to be built at Ashton General Hospital in the near future, which would provide excellent facilities and opportunities for pupil midwives. It seemed like the perfect opening for me, but I wanted to be absolutely sure it would be the right move. After all, this was a major decision for me. I had worked very hard to get this far, and I didn't want to take the wrong path now. I had thoroughly enjoyed St Mary's, and just thinking about it warmed my heart. I could still smell the cosy scent of talcum powder and sweet milk in the air, and if I closed my eyes I could feel the babies in my arms, snug and content, snuffling as I rocked them to sleep. What if Ashton wasn't the same? I'd regret the decision very much.

I made an appointment to see Mrs Ingham at St Mary's one afternoon to canvas her opinion. She told me Ashton General was a friendly hospital where she thought I would fit in perfectly thanks to my 'equable' temperament, and promised to give me a fine reference. I was chuffed to bits. I valued Mrs Ingham's opinion highly and this was just what I wanted to hear. With Mr Tate's help I wrote a letter of application a few days later, addressed to Miss Ripley, the Matron of Ashton General Hospital. The wheels were set in motion, and I could almost feel them rolling beneath my feet. This was incredibly exciting. My dream of becoming a midwife was within touching distance now.

On 27 August 1969 Miss Bell asked Mrs Ingham to provide a reference for me, and on 9 September Mrs Ingham filled in a questionnaire about the 'obstetric nurse training course' I had completed at St Mary's, which was then sent to Miss Ripley, my prospective new matron. I never saw the documents at the time, but I know these dates now because in 2008, when I tried to retire, I was presented with a copy of the original questionnaire. It had lain in my file for more than forty years, and this is what Mrs Ingham wrote about me:

1. State of Health and amount of sick leave: 'Apparently healthy. No such leave during above course.'
2. Temper and Disposition: 'A very pleasing personality. Equable temperament.'
3. Reliability: 'Always reliable and punctual.'
4. Manner and appearance: 'An attractive girl. Always well "groomed".'
5. Intelligence and Education: 'An intelligent girl. Grammar School Education. Written work and record keeping well above average standard.'
6.. General remarks: 'This girl was a most satisfactory student whilst undergoing the above mentioned training. She was extremely interested in her work and her nurse–patient relationship was excellent.'

I remember asking my mum what the word 'equable' meant after I first heard Mrs Ingham use it when I went to St Mary's to ask for her opinion on my career.

'It means you are level-headed and not easily disturbed,' Mum told me.

We were out shopping for my wedding dress, and were walking though to the plush bridal department at Marshall & Snelgrove in Manchester.

'Look, Mum!' I said excitedly. 'Look at this one! It's absolutely gorgeous!'

The dazzling white dress was displayed on a glamorous mannequin right in the middle of the floor, and I was thrilled to see there was the most beautiful long, lace veil floating behind it.

'Can I try it on?'

Mum turned over the price tag to reveal that the dress cost the extravagant sum of £50 – not far off two months of my wages.

'Go on then,' she smiled indulgently. 'So much for being "equable", though, Linda!'

The dress fitted perfectly and I was very touched that Mum was more than happy to pay for it. It wasn't about the money; I was delighted that she was clearly supportive of my decision to marry Graham, and that she wanted to push the boat out for me.

The next few months passed in a whirl. In the September I received a certificate through the post telling me I had passed my exams and qualified as an SRN nurse. The certificate itself was disappointingly plain and delivered without a fanfare, but what it represented was incredibly important to me. As a qualified SRN I was now able to dispense with the three stripes of white bias binding on my sleeve that marked me out as a third-year student. Instead, I would now have the honour of wearing the MRI 'strings' on my hat, a green belt around my waist and the prized MRI bronze penny on my dress. This meant the world to me. All I needed to do now was complete my obligatory three months' work at the MRI post-qualifying, which would enable me to receive my official MRI nursing certificate in December.

Along with about twenty-five others from our intake, Nessa, Anne, Jo and I were all invited to Miss Bell's office one morning to receive our penny. While waiting outside to be called in individually, we hugged and giggled like little girls.

'All this for a bronze penny!' Anne joked. 'I think we deserve more than a penny after what we've been through!'

We laughed, knowing that, like the rest of us, she couldn't wait to get her hands on the shiny medal. It depicted the Good Samaritan and, in Latin, bore Jesus' words *Vade et tu fac similiter*, meaning 'Go, and do thou likewise.' We'd seen it many times, pinned proudly to the uniforms of other nurses, and we could scarcely believe we were finally joining their ranks as fully-fledged staff nurses.

'Congratulations, Nurse Lawton,' Miss Bell said, shaking my hand when it was finally my turn to step up to her desk. I smiled broadly as she handed me my shining penny. 'You have worked hard. Well done!'

'Thank you,' I said. 'Thank you for …'

'No need to thank me,' she interrupted briskly. '*You* have done this. Good luck!'

The next stop was the sewing room where we all eagerly claimed a brand new green belt that fastened with Velcro around our waists, and finally got our hands on two white 'strings' each. A home sister showed us how to attach the strings to our hats using white kirby grips before securing them correctly in a neat bow under the chin.

'I can't move in this!' Jo complained, pulling open her too-tight bow as we huddled in a corner to practise.

'I know, this is such a nuisance,' Anne niggled as her strings disappeared into a fold underneath her generous chin. 'Wearing these makes you feel like a puppet!'

With that she jerked her head from side to side, as if an invisible puppeteer were manoeuvring her. 'Thunderbirds are GO!' she mocked. 'Or should that be MRI nurses are GO?'

'Yes m'Lady!' Jo retorted jokily, though she was still struggling with her bow and pulling a disgruntled face.

Nessa and I exchanged knowing glances. For all their moaning, we both knew that Anne and Jo were tickled pink, just as we were. We'd made it, and at long last we were in the clique. As Sister Mary Francis might say, we weren't just nurses; we were MRI nurses, no less!

'Does anybody know how Cynthia is getting on?' Anne asked as we strode out of the sewing room in our new attire, shoulders back and heads held high.

'Do you know, you read my mind,' I replied. 'I was just thinking about Cynthia. I went to see her a few days ago. She was sitting up in bed, knitting a scarf and looking very pale, but her operation has been a great success. She told me she's very pleased for us all for passing our exams, and not to worry about her. She's going to catch up next year, so she'll soon get her penny.'

'Good for her,' Jo said. 'I'm not sure I'd have managed to carry on if I were in her shoes.'

We all nodded in agreement. 'She's remarkable,' I said. I'd learned that the reason Cynthia stitched all her own clothes by hand was because she came from a very poor family and her mother couldn't afford to buy a sewing machine, let alone new clothes. I'd admired Cynthia's tenacity, even before she became ill.

I couldn't help wondering how Janice was getting on, wherever she was, not to mention Linda, who had only written once since her departure, with very little news. Thinking about them both, as well as Cynthia, made me count my blessings. I touched my penny and said a silent little prayer, thanking God for the life I had.

Within weeks I learned that my application to become a pupil midwife at Ashton General had been processed and I was to attend an interview in early December. Should I secure the position, I would start on 1 January 1970 and I would earn £100 a month. This sounded like a fortune compared to my current salary, although of course I was used to having my accommodation fees deducted at source, so in reality it wasn't as huge an increase as it seemed. In any case, I was far more interested in the position than the salary, and I was incredibly excited to be one step closer to achieving my ambition.

Everything was happening so fast. My heart was packed with emotions, and I took out my diary and unloaded some of my feelings onto its pages.

'Life is changing,' I wrote, under the date 28 September 1969.

It seems a lifetime ago that I arrived at the MRI, frightened and homesick, yet it also seems like only yesterday when I first put on my nurse's uniform. Isn't that strange? Am I ready to train to become a midwife? Yes, I am! I will miss my friends here, but I am ready to leave now. I can't wait to get married – and I really want to be a pupil midwife!!

Graham and I married on 22 November 1969 at St Michael and All Angels Church in Ashton. Being so close to finally finishing at the MRI really put an extra shine on my day. Seeing Graham standing at the altar waiting for me, I felt like the luckiest girl in the world. In that moment, I had it all. Not only was I marrying my handsome soulmate, but I had a wonderful career at my fingertips. Any doubts that I might not be accepted as a pupil midwife left me that day and I was filled with optimism about my future, or our future, as it now was.

My old school friend Sue, by now a qualified teacher, was my bridesmaid, along with Graham's teenage sister, Barbara. It was a very cold day and they shivered in their deep turquoise dresses as they attended to my gown at the back of the church, making sure my long veil and train were sitting just so. I felt the high lace collar snug around my neck as I swallowed deeply, savouring the moment when Dad took my arm and began to walk me slowly towards my husband to be.

I could almost feel myself growing up just that little bit more as I took each step towards Graham. My head was held high and my heartbeat was steady and strong, secure in the knowledge I was making my parents proud, and making my way successfully in the world.

I remember feeling giddy with happiness when the Church of England minister declared us man and wife, and I also recall being delighted it didn't rain as we made our way to the local Masonic Hall for our wedding reception.

My mum had made most of the arrangements, and the majority of the fifty invited guests were long-standing family friends and relatives. I didn't ask any of my nursing friends, as this part of my life seemed so separate from my working life. Besides, in those days it wasn't really the done thing to have a big knees-up with your peers.

We ate minestrone soup with a warm roll and a curl of butter, followed by roast beef and Yorkshire pudding with thick gravy, and rounded off with lemon meringue pie. Afterwards Mrs Cox, one of my parents' friends who frequently came to our house to play cards, played the piano and sang loudly, which encouraged several couples to shuffle around the dance floor to tunes like 'Can't Take My Eyes Off You' by Frankie Valli and 'Green, Green Grass of Home' by Tom Jones.

'Congratulations on becoming Mrs Linda Buckley,' an elderly colleague of my father's said jovially as he chinked my glass of champagne and admired my gleaming wedding band. 'Tell me, are you going to give up work now you're a newly married lady?'

I burst out laughing. 'Certainly not,' I replied. 'I'm planning to train as a midwife!'

'Good heavens!' he remarked in mock surprise. 'In my day women had babies themselves when they got married, they didn't set about delivering other people's!'

'It's very nearly 1970 and, luckily for me, times have changed!' I responded with amusement.

It was one of those moments when the words that come out of your mouth strike an unexpected chord. This one resonated throughout my whole body. There I was, dressed in my beautiful wedding gown with my new husband looking resplendent across the room in his dark grey morning suit, chatting contentedly to our guests. Our new home was ready for us to move in to and there, sitting tantalisingly in a mahogany letter rack on our new hall table, lay the key to my future: the all-important letter detailing my imminent interview at Ashton General Hospital. I felt very fortunate indeed.

Graham and I would have children one day, I hoped. We'd discussed it before we married, of course, and had agreed we'd like to start a family in a few years. I was twenty-one and he was twenty, so we had time on our side. I imagined we'd be in our mid-twenties when we became parents; that sounded about right. For the time being Graham was ploughing all his money into his business, Buckley Vending Supplies, and we still had plenty of work to do on our new home. We were in no rush to become parents, and we would take precautions for the time being.

When Graham carried me over the threshold and took me to bed for the first time, I pictured all my doubts and fears falling away, scattering and disappearing into the confetti-sprinkled carpet. We had a short honeymoon in York, chosen as I could only get a week off work and it wasn't too far to travel, or too expensive. One of the highlights for me was visiting York Minster, which brought back fond memories of being at my convent school. When you have been educated by nuns I don't think their influence ever leaves you. I recall sitting quietly in a pew at the back beside Graham and feeling deeply peaceful and very happy. If God was guiding me, I was pleased with where He had brought me so far in my life. I was where I wanted to be, and I felt thankful. To this day, though I am not a regular churchgoer, I still believe in God and am comforted by the thought He may be up there somewhere, watching over me and my patients.

Back at the MRI the week after our honeymoon I was once again called to Miss Bell's office, where I was handed my MRI certificate. This was the final certificate, and the one I had been waiting for. It officially recognised that, as well as being an SRN, I was an MRI nurse too. I had looked forward to this day, and I studied the certificate with immense pride in my heart.

Emblazoned with the words 'United Manchester Hospitals School of Nursing' the certificate proclaimed in elaborate script:

This Certificate is awarded to Linda Mary Lawton for efficiency in Medical and Surgical Nursing as proved by work done in the wards over a period of three years and three months and after examination.

It was signed by both the Chairman of the Board of Governors and the Chairman of the Medical Executive Committee, as well as Constance Biddulph, the Principal of United Manchester Hospitals School of Nursing. The date on the bottom was 5 December 1969. My three years and three months of training and work at the MRI slipped into the past, right there. What mattered now was using this piece of paper to set me on the road to carving out a future for myself as a midwife.

I couldn't wait to get home, see Graham and show him my longed-for certificate. My journey back seemed to take forever, as since moving into our new home together I'd taken to travelling in and out of Manchester by bus. It was far from ideal, and each day involved a lot of messing about. I had to leave the house more than an hour before my shift started in the morning, and on the return journey I often had to change buses and wait around in the cold, shivering under my NHS gabardine. I never thought I'd say it, but living in the nurses' home had been a godsend in many ways. As a student I would never have coped with a daily commute on top of everything else, and the thought of applying to St Mary's should I fail to secure a place at Ashton now seemed completely untenable.

I was exhausted when I finally put my key in the door, and I almost fell onto the burgundy floral carpet in our hallway that evening.

'How's my little nurse?' Graham called jovially. He was sitting on one of our dark red Draylon-covered bowl-shaped armchairs, drinking a mug of steaming tea and watching *Dad's Army* on our small Rediffusion television. Our new budgerigar, whom we'd named Billy Buckley, flapped around his cage in the corner of the room, and a gold-coloured carriage clock we'd received as a wedding present, which now took pride of place on the brick mantelpiece, told me it was just gone 7.30 p.m. That meant I'd been out of the house for almost thirteen hours.

'Tired!' I said, an image of Jo, Anne and Nessa flashing through my mind. They'd waved to me at the bus stop more than an hour earlier, having eaten together in the dining room before heading to their flat. They'd have been home by 6.30 p.m. at the latest, I reckoned.

'I'd have picked you up after work, you know, if you'd let me.'

'I know, but I can't expect you to do that every night, and you have your own job to do without running around after me ...'

'I was thinking,' Graham said. 'My business is going well and we can afford to buy a few new things.'

'Like what?'

'A colour television?' he smiled, looking at me hopefully.

This didn't excite me in the least and I told him so, rather begrudgingly. I rarely had time to watch television, let alone worry about whether I was watching in black and white or colour. Besides, we didn't have any savings after the expense of buying our first home, and only the week before I'd gratefully accepted my mum's offer that she would buy our Christmas turkey for us.

I made my way down the hall to the kitchen, ready to start cooking the dinner, thinking that I wasn't very impressed with this set-up. I had my interview at Ashton in a few days and I felt worn out, but I accepted that now I was a wife it was my duty to cook for my new husband, whatever time I got in from work.

'There's a wimberry pie for pudding,' Graham called after me. 'Your mum dropped it in earlier.'

I pushed open the kitchen door, stopped and gaped. There in front of me, glinting in the middle of the lino, was a shiny grey Honda 50 moped.

'Like it?' Graham asked, looming behind me and spinning me round so he could see the surprised look in my eye.

'Oh yes!' I grinned. 'Is it for me? It's absolutely brilliant!'

'Thought you would. You don't need to take lessons or a test, just wear "L" plates. It's very easy to ride. I thought it would help you get around.'

He had splashed out £26 on it, and I was beyond thrilled. 'I really hope I get that job,' I said. 'Just think, I could scoot to work in no time at all. Thank you, Graham! Thank you so much!'

'What about a colour TV as well …?" he asked, but I could tell from the mischievous look on his face he was only teasing me with that one.

'No!' I said. 'We've barely got enough furniture yet! You've really spoiled me, Graham. You couldn't have got me anything better.' It was too late to venture out that night and I was tired out anyhow, but I really looked forward to trying it out the next morning.

When the day of my interview finally arrived I tried to play it cool, even though I was flapping around the house more than Billy Buckley in his cage.

'Are you nervous?' Graham asked as I fixed and re-fixed my hair in a bun and charged up and down the stairs with different coats, seeing which one looked best over my smart navy-blue skirt, pressed blouse and fine-knit cardigan.

'Not really,' I fibbed. 'I know I stand a good chance of getting this post. I've got the right qualifications and there's a place for me if they think I can do it. It's not as if hundreds of people are fighting over the job.'

All this was true, but of course there were no guarantees. I still had to impress Miss Sefton. She had the power to end my dream this very day. I had to prove I was right for this role, and that I wanted it with all my heart.

In the event, my interview turned out to be a breeze, after Mrs Ingham appeared unexpectedly and introduced me enthusiastically to the interview panel as 'my little obstetric nurse'. I discovered Mrs Ingham was an occasional visiting tutor at Ashton's Maternity Unit, giving lectures to pupil midwives. I really hoped I'd be in her class one day.

To my relief, Miss Sefton, Head of Midwifery, and Miss O'Neil, Deputy Head of Midwifery, both followed Mrs Ingham's lead, welcoming me so warmly I felt as if I were practically one of the family.

Miss Sefton was small and smartly dressed in a burgundy dress with a mandarin collar. She pursed her lips as she spoke, which made her look strict and posh, but she was also very friendly, even congratulating me on my marriage. Miss O'Neil was younger and dressed in a grey uniform, and she too seemed very pleasant. Compared to meeting Miss Morgan at the MRI, it was as easy as pie.

Despite the convivial atmosphere, I still sat bolt upright throughout the interview and took care to speak clearly and give sensible, considered answers. It wasn't difficult, as most questions were about whether or not I was happy to do shift work, attend lectures outside working hours and do night duty – all of which I expected and was perfectly willing to agree to.

At the end of the questioning Miss Sefton announced that she would like to offer me a position as a pupil midwife, and that a letter would be in the post. She then went on to give details of pay, holidays and so forth, which I was too over-whelmed to take in fully.

'Thank you!' I beamed as all three women bid me a cheer-ful goodbye.

I could scarcely believe it, and I don't think I really did until a formal letter arrived in the post a week later, officially offer-ing me the position of pupil midwife. To say it was a dream come true is an understatement; I was beside myself with happiness and brimming with anticipation. I was actually going to train as a midwife. Me, Linda Buckley! Imagine that! What's more, now I could relax a little and enjoy my last few weeks at the MRI.

With Christmas just around the corner, the hospital was all decked out with tinsel and paper chains. There was always a competition for the best-decorated ward, and the sisters took tremendous pride in striving to make theirs the winner. On Christmas Day itself, the consultant always carved the turkey on the ward, and the registrar would dress as Santa. The lights were dimmed when carol singers visited, and the patients usually joined in with hymns, singing from their beds.

We always tried to get as many patients as possible home for Christmas Day, though past experience taught me that many preferred to stay in hospital, especially if they had nobody at home to share the day with. I'd worked the past three Christmases, and I always said it was the only day of the year you could let yourself go at the MRI, if only just a little bit.

This year, I had the misfortune of working for Sister Bridie, who appeared to be the only member of staff in the entire hospital not to have joined in the Christmas spirit. For a start, she was the only one not to have attached a piece of tinsel or sprig of holly to her uniform.

'Lawton, see to Mrs Strongintharm,' she ordered, her voice pitted with irritation and sounding more shrill and Irish than ever. I considered asking her to call me Buckley now I was married, but decided it wasn't worth the bother.

I'd never heard the name 'Strongintharm' before, but this was indeed the lady's name. Mrs Strongintharm was sitting up in bed, merrily singing 'Jingle Bells' out of tune, at the top of her voice. Her jolly disposition was totally at odds with the dismal din blasting from her lips. The woman in the next bed was complaining, 'Ooh for heaven's sake, put a sock in it, Mrs S!' but Mrs Strongintharm was too busy enjoying herself to listen, and carried on regardless.

Mrs Strongintharm had a huge bulbous body with skinny legs that stuck out beneath her as she sat jiggling away on the bed. I wondered how on earth such stick-like limbs could support her boulder of a body when she stood up. She was clicking her fingers now as she wobbled her body from side to side in time to the music, her face twinkling as gaily as the brightly lit Christmas tree in the middle of the ward. I could see that she was one of those patients who was more than happy to spend Christmas in hospital, and I didn't want to upset her.

'Mrs Strongintharm, Sister has asked me to have a word,' I said softly.

'Oh what fun it is to ride on a one-horse open sleigh!' she trilled joyfully, totally ignoring me.

'It's time for your medication, and I think you may be disturbing some of the other patients,' I appealed. This time I spoke as loudly and plainly as I could without sounding rude, for Mrs Strongintharm was belting out the song with even more gusto than before.

'Dashing through the snow, laughing all the way …' she continued, starting to conduct an imaginary orchestra with her short, swinging arms.

It was already a surreal scene, and I suddenly found myself watching in what felt like slow motion as Mrs Strongintharm lunged dramatically to the left, lost her balance, rolled off the bed and hit the floor with a thump. I made a grab for her in shock.

'For pity's sake!' I heard a gruff voice shout. It was Dennis, the male charge nurse I'd worked with in Casualty. 'Take her legs!' he snapped as he hooked his hands under Mrs Strongintharm's armpits and heaved and rolled her back into bed with impressive skill and speed.

'Thanks, Dennis,' I said later, once we'd checked her over and found no harm had been done. 'I don't know what I would have done if you hadn't been passing.'

'It's all right,' he winked. 'Lucky I had some parcels to deliver up here. At least the bump shut her up, eh? Strongintharm but weak in th' head you'll have to call that one from now on!'

Sister Bridie appeared soon afterwards. 'I don't know what you did to Mrs Strongintharm but she's behaved herself perfectly since you dealt with her,' she remarked. 'You've come on in leaps and bounds, Lawton, haven't you?'

'The MRI has taught me well, Sister Bridie,' I said diplomatically.

'It has indeed,' she said. 'But take that silly tinsel off your dress. We're here to work, not to decorate the place.'

As I untied the skinny strip of red glitter that was wrapped around my fob watch and slid it in my pocket, Sister Bridie eyed me approvingly.

'Good luck in your new post, Lawton,' she said with a dry smile.

'Thank you,' I replied. 'I'm looking forward to it very much indeed.'

On my last day I slipped away quietly. I had already said my goodbyes to Nessa, Anne and Jo, which was easy as we'd promised to keep in touch and were all staying locally. I was glad to be leaving, to be honest, and I didn't imagine I would miss anything at all about the MRI besides my friends. It had served me well, standing me in good stead for the next stage of my career, and now it was time to move on.

I changed out of my uniform for the last time, folded it up and placed it neatly in a laundry bag. A feeling of sadness took me by surprise, and I wondered whether perhaps I had been too busy to consider how momentous the day actually was. I had removed the bronze penny from my uniform before taking it off, and now I looked at it with admiration and squeezed it in my palm. I'd always have it to remind me of my training, and I pledged to myself that I would always strive to maintain the high standards of the MRI, wherever I worked in future.

Chapter Nine

*'To qualify as a midwife you'll need to
deliver forty babies in ten months'*

I fired up my moped and set off for Ashton General Hospital
with adrenaline zipping about inside me. It was early in the
morning on Thursday 1 January 1970, and at last I was starting my new post as a pupil midwife.

Cutting through the bitterly cold morning air and circling
Stamford Park Lake as I neared the hospital, I remembered
how I'd told Graham the interview here just a few weeks
earlier was as 'easy as pie'. The phrase stuck in my throat
now. It reminded me of the blasé attitude I'd had towards
the MRI after my very first visit as a naïve eighteen-year-
old. Though I was giddy with excitement, I shivered inside
my thick winter coat, suddenly wondering if I would rue
my words and find the daily grind much harder than I
expected.

I had been told in my job offer letter to report to Sister Kelly
on Ward 16 of the Maternity Unit, in the part of the hospital
known as 'The Lake'. It was a very old building, originally a
workhouse, and it was separated from the main Infirmary by
Fountain Street. As I approached the hospital I suddenly felt
daunted by its vast dimensions. I was used to the tall yet relatively compact MRI building, but this hospital sprawled
outwards instead of rising neatly upwards. I'd never noticed

how big it was before, but then again I'd never had to think about navigating my way around it before.

Apart from my interview, I'd only ever visited the hospital on two previous occasions. One was several years earlier when I went to visit my Auntie Mary, who was having treatment in the Infirmary, and the other time was when I had my appendix out at the age of fourteen, also in the Infirmary.

As I secured my moped to the railings at the side of the hospital and looked at window after window carved in the wide red-brick walls, I had a vivid flashback to lying in my hospital bed as a worried teenager, having just been visited by my mum and dad. I longed to go home with them and wanted to cry when they said goodbye, then all of a sudden they popped up outside the window next to my bed, smiling and waving and mouthing 'See you later, Linda!' through the glass. It really cheered me up, and I recalled how I clutched my newly stitched wound and laughed.

Now I could almost feel a pain in my abdomen all over again, but it had nothing to do with a burst appendix, just plain nerves. As I entered the main reception and headed along a wide corridor, a pleasant, sweet smell penetrated my nostrils. I noticed the walls were coated with speckled cream paint that was peeling in parts, and nurses in blue dresses rushed along, waving and saying 'Happy New Year!' to everybody but me – or so it seemed. The smell reminded me of pear drops, I thought to myself, and I liked it.

I didn't have my uniform yet, and as I made my way upstairs to the Maternity Unit on the first floor I felt quite insignificant, invisible even, in mufti. For a moment I wished I was in my MRI uniform, but then instinctively felt glad I wasn't. I didn't want anybody to think that I thought I was a cut above the rest, showing off about coming from a fancy teaching hospital.

The uniform here was more modern and didn't look quite as grand as the one I was used to. It was made of a similar sort of stiff fabric as the MRI dress, but was in a denim blue, and had a less flamboyant apron that simply pinned up onto the bust instead of crossing over the shoulders. I was pleased to see I would still wear detachable cuffs over my short sleeves, and wondered if the nurses here called them 'frillies' as we did at the MRI. I imagined they did.

'Ah, pleased to meet yer, Linda!' Sister Kelly grinned as I found her in a kitchen beside her office off Ward 16. 'Sit yerself down here and have a drink of hot orange. You must be frozen to the bone!'

I obliged, smiling involuntarily at the sound of her strong Irish accent. It was even more pronounced than Sister Bridie's, but it didn't grate on my nerves as hers had. In fact, I found Sister Kelly's voice instantly endearing.

I shook her large, outstretched hand and felt my fingers crushed roughly together inside her broad palm. I smiled as she turned to switch on the kettle that was already puffing out steam, no doubt from the recent brew that was sitting on the worktop beside her. A second later I felt the smile freeze on my face as I watched her give her left buttock a mighty scratch through the back of her navy-blue dress, before reaching down her front to reposition her bra and its contents. She then gave her bust a good long scratch, too. I was flabbergasted.

It was at this point that I also registered the fact that Sister Kelly's uniform had several stains on it, and she was wearing a scruffy knitted liberty bodice that was visible under her dress. Protruding from under her sister's cap were straggles of what appeared to be quite greasy hair.

I'd never seen anything like this at the MRI, and I tried not to stare. What would Sister Craddock think of Sister Kelly? I couldn't help wondering. The phrase 'cleanliness is next to godliness' would not be far from her lips, I was sure of that.

'Get that down yer before yer catch yer death, while I tell yer what's what around here,' Sister Kelly instructed kindly, leading me into her office.

I'd never had hot orange before and I didn't really fancy it, but I did as I was told and sipped the steaming liquid, which was served in a heavy mug that had a chip on the rim and was stained brown inside. Despite her somewhat off-putting appearance, Sister Kelly exuded the most amazing warmth, and I found myself very comfortable in her company as I listened intently to what I had in store.

Ward 16, I learned, was a postnatal ward for normal deliveries. The women here had no complications, and would typically stay with us for two days after giving birth. For the first two months it would be my duty to assist with the general running of the ward by making beds, caring for the new mothers, feeding, bathing and changing their babies and generally helping out in the way I had done on my placement at St Mary's. My midwifery training would not commence officially until March, when I would attend lectures with tutors, one of whom was Miss Sefton. Mrs Ingham would also put in the odd appearance to give talks, which I was pleased to hear.

Sister Kelly barely drew breath before explaining that she would then 'lose me' to Ward 18, which was for women who'd had forceps, Caesarean or other more complicated deliveries. I would also do short placements on the antenatal ward, labour ward, the neonatal unit and in the antenatal clinic. All of this would take me up to June, and would constitute Part One of my midwifery training.

As I was a qualified SRN and had done my obstetric nurse training, I only had to complete a ten-month course. The subsequent six months that made up Part Two would see me venturing out into the community with an experienced community midwife called Mrs May Tattersall, who would be my mentor. If all went to plan, I would be a qualified midwife by December 1970.

'I know it's an awful lot to take in!' Sister Kelly laughed. 'But I've heard yer good with numbers, Linda, and yer'd need to be for the next ting I'm going to tell yer.'

I smiled obligingly, not wanting to tell Sister Kelly that I'd already been given much of this information in the letter offering me the post. She was clearly enjoying being my mother hen, and I was quite enjoying being clucked over in her cosy office.

'This is the important bit, my dear. To qualify as a midwife you'll need to deliver forty babies in ten months, from March to December in your case. Forty sounds like an immense number, doesn't it?' she chuckled.

I nodded, mentally calculating that meant at least one a week, and that's if I started on day one of my training course.

'On top of that you have to witness six breech births, six forceps deliveries and six Caesarean sections, but don't you worry ya'self one bit. This daft old hippy ting of wanting to have babies at home is changing, mark my words. We're getting busier by the day in here. The bigwigs in London want more women to give birth in hospital, didn't ya know? Better for the infant mortality figures, that's what they reckon. You won't have any trouble at all, Linda, and when I say you have to deliver the babies, I don't mean all by yerself. And don't forget, you can always come and talk to me if anyting is botherin' yer. I'm always ready for a chat. I like a chat, so I do!'

Sister Kelly handed me my new uniform and directed me to the female changing rooms on the ground floor. I was relieved to get changed, as I didn't want to stand out as the new girl in mufti. I put the uniform on quickly, checking myself just once in the mirror. The denim blue dress had a navy-coloured belt that fitted comfortably around my waist and was secured with Velcro on top of my apron. I wore black stockings and suspenders and flat black leather lace-up shoes, and carried scissors in my pocket that were attached by a chain to my belt. On the left-hand side of my chest I pinned a new fob watch that I'd received as a gift from Sue's mum, and I added the detachable cuffs that I would soon discover were indeed referred to as 'frillies' here too. I felt a million dollars as I stepped back out onto the corridor and started to make my way upstairs to Ward 16.

My head was in the clouds a little as I tried to retrace my steps. I was thinking how strange it was that I felt at home there so quickly. The whole atmosphere seemed so friendly, so much more relaxed than at the MRI. The pleasant pear-drop smell was certainly better than the omnipresent smell of powerful cleaning fluid and disinfectant I was used to. I could detect the scent of talcum powder and fresh laundry in the air, too, as I walked dreamily along. That, coupled with the smell of newborn babies, seemed to be what gave the pear-drop smell.

'Have you never heard of contraception?'

I nearly jumped out of my uniform. The question boomed very loudly from behind a thin screen, as if blasted through a loudspeaker, and was quickly followed by the quivering sound of a young girl saying meekly, 'I'm sorry, Dr Franklin, really I am.'

I wanted to stop in my tracks and listen, but I kept walking, even though I realised I was heading in the wrong direction.

'How stupid can you be?' the gruff doctor raged, his voice somehow sounding louder the further away I walked. 'We'll have to bloody well sterilise you!'

Clearly, I was passing through antenatal, and I deduced this must be a poor young girl who had found herself pregnant by accident, obviously not for the first time. This Dr Franklin sounded like an angry headmaster chastising a naughty pupil. How terribly sad for the pregnant girl, and how dreadfully embarrassing to be told off so publicly. Surely he must know the whole ward could hear him ranting?

'There he goes again, cheeky devil!' a nurse walking behind me mumbled to a colleague. I turned to see them raise their eyes to the heavens before disappearing into a side room. I carried on, eventually finding my way back to Ward 16 via a maze of unfamiliar corridors. A friendly staff nurse called Margaret Mulligan greeted me.

'I'm told we're on bed-making together,' she said. 'Do you like The Fivepenny Piece?'

'Oh yes,' I said. 'I've seen them quite a few times in the Broadoak Hotel.'

'I think we all have!!' Margaret smiled. 'Us nurses must be their biggest fans. We sing their songs all the time while we make the beds. Helps pass the time.'

With that she led me to the linen cupboard, gave me a pile of sheets, blankets and pillowcases and proceeded towards the far end of Ward 16. It was a Nightingale ward, yet it seemed very different to the ones I was used to.

'Hello, Nurses!' a couple of ladies chirped as we passed their beds. Their babies were lying quietly beside them in their small linen hammock cots, and the two proud new mums were chatting to each other about a knitting pattern in a magazine.

'I'll bring it over to yours when I've finished with it,' the first woman said.

'Thanks, Lottie, love. I'll look forward to that. We'll have a cuppa and a chin-wag.'

'That's lucky,' I commented to Margaret. 'Fancy two friends ending up in neighbouring beds.'

'Oh, they weren't friends before,' Margaret smiled, 'but they've never stopped jawing since they met. Often happens in here. Having a baby on the same day seems to bind people together like nothing else. Nice, isn't it?'

I nodded. That's what was so different about this ward. It had an incredibly homely, friendly feel to it, even more welcoming than at St Mary's, I felt.

Margaret started singing The Fivepenny Piece's eponymous signature tune as we set to work, encouraging me to join in. Before I knew it we'd made five beds and also sung 'Mountain Climber' and 'Stories from the Wishing Well'.

By now a couple of patients were humming and singing along, and one lady was walking up and down the ward, rocking her baby in her arms in time to our music.

'Oooh, it is a giggle in here,' Lottie exclaimed. 'Makes you want to come back!'

Several women groaned playfully at her suggestion. 'How could you even *think* about having another baby?' one exhausted-looking young woman winced. 'I never want to have marital relations again, let alone another baby!'

'You'll change your mind soon enough, love,' Lottie chuckled. 'Most of us do, more fool us!'

When the steaming lunch trolley arrived, twelve of the ladies seated themselves around the long wooden dining table in the middle of the ward, leaving their babies lying in their cots. If it wasn't for the fact the women were all in their twenties and dressed in candlewick dressing gowns and slippers, they would have looked for all the world like a group of giddy classmates waiting for their school dinner.

'I 'ope it's not blessed tripe or liver,' Lottie's pal Bessie hissed loudly behind her hand.

'Blinkin' 'eck, don't say that!' Lottie sniggered. 'Makes me come over all queasy. I'm still recoverin' from the sight of that placenta!'

The whole table erupted in a collective chorus of complaints. 'Stop it, you'll put us off us dinner!' 'Don't be so crude!' 'How could you!' 'Ooooh, don't make me laugh, you'll 'ave me stitches falling out!'

The sound of Sister Kelly's heavy footsteps approaching made the women stop talking and laughing as they looked up to see who was coming. I think they knew better than I did that Sister Kelly wasn't strict and liked nothing better than having a chat and a cuppa at every opportunity. Still, all the patients treated her with respect, cutting out their cheeky banter and behaving themselves impeccably in her presence.

Two pupil midwives accompanied Sister Kelly and the trio began to serve up the luncheon with some ceremony. While one nurse held out each white porcelain plate, the other used an industrial-sized spoon to dollop a generous helping of boiled potatoes then a mound of steaming cabbage onto it. Meanwhile, at the head of the trolley, Sister Kelly brandished a giant fork, which she used to skewer thin slices of meat laid out on a stainless steel platter, before depositing them portion by portion alongside the bland potatoes and soggy cabbage.

Once the ladies each had a plateful in front of them, one of the midwives circled the dining table with a heavy jug and poured thick, lumpy puddles of gravy on every meal in precise rotation, never once asking if anybody actually wanted it.

'Enjoy your meal now, ladies!' Sister Kelly instructed merrily before thumping back down the ward, retrieving her underwear from between her buttocks as she did so. Nobody seemed to notice or, if they did, her habits didn't appear to offend or surprise them.

'Who was it said she was a farmer's daughter?' Lottie whispered loudly once Sister Kelly was out of earshot.

'I can't remember who said it, but it's as plain as the nose on your face, isn't it?' Bessie replied jovially. 'The way she wields that serving fork, you can just imagine her pitching it into a bale of hay and tossing it into the back of a tractor!'

'How do you get your deliveries?' I asked Margaret when we went for a tea break later. I was still wondering how I would manage to clock up forty in ten months.

'Oh, it's a doddle,' she said. 'There's a bell in each delivery room, and every time there's a birth imminent the midwife will ring it, and any pupil midwives working on the maternity wards needing to clock up a birth can run in. Even catching the baby at the last minute counts towards your forty deliveries.'

'What about the complicated ones, the forceps, breech and Caesareans?'

'You only have to witness those, of course, as the doctors are in charge,' Margaret said. 'Sometimes you'll just get lucky. We have no way of telling in advance whether a normal delivery is going to turn into something more complicated. I've delivered twins to several women who thought they were only having one baby. We palpate the abdomen and use the Pinard ear trumpet in antenatal clinic to feel and listen for more than one heartbeat, but it certainly isn't a foolproof way of knowing for sure how many babies are in there, as you'll no doubt find out. In my experience one twin has a habit of coming out bottom first, and that's how I got to witness all of my breech births.'

When I think back to that conversation I can scarcely believe how we managed without the routine ultrasound scans we rely on today. Now, it is practically unheard of not to detect multiple babies in advance, and in the vast majority of cases the woman is booked in for a Caesarean to limit the risk of complications during delivery.

'For forceps and Caesarean births, you'd need a crystal ball to predict them,' Margaret went on. 'Sometimes the smoothest of births suddenly becomes an emergency and, before you know it, it's theatre gowns and general anaesthetic at the double, or the consultant is wielding the Kielland forceps. Needless to say, nobody comes in here planning a Caesarean section or a forceps delivery. Even with multiple births and breech babies, we encourage all the women to have as natural a delivery as possible.'

'Don't women who know they are having twins or a breech ever ask if they can have a Caesarean?' I asked, wide-eyed.

'No!' Margaret smiled. 'The women never ask anything. We tell them what's what and they never question us. I swear, if a midwife told a pregnant woman to jump, her reply would be "How high?" every time.'

Margaret laughed and I joined in.

'Hey,' she asked, still giggling and with a mischievous glint in her eye. 'I see you're married, Linda. Tell me, at your interview, did Mrs Sefton ask you what sort of contraception you used?'

'No!' I stammered. 'Why would she?'

'She must have liked the look of you. She usually gives pupil midwives the third degree. Poor Dorothy was asked that question outright and was so taken aback she just answered, saying she was taking the Pill. She told me she would never even discuss such a thing with her own mother! Apparently Miss Sefton looked over her reading glasses and said, "I'm very glad to hear it. I like my nurses to be *responsible*." Poor Dorothy came out of the office with her face as red as a tomato!'

I liked Margaret a lot. I felt I could ask her anything, and I had a feeling I would be picking her brains many more times in the months to come. As we walked back to the ward I described to her how I'd taken a wrong turning earlier and overheard Dr Franklin shouting at a young girl.

'I couldn't believe my ears,' I said. 'I've never heard a doctor speak to a patient like that before.'

'You'd better get used to it,' she sighed. 'He's well known for having the most dreadful bedside manner. The thing about maternity is that the patients are not actually ill; they are simply pregnant. As I'm sure you know, consultants can be bullish at the best of times. The fact they are not dealing with the sick seems to make them think they can get away with absolute murder. Don't worry too much about Dr Franklin, though; he's got a soft heart underneath all the bluster.'

As we approached Ward 16 after our tea break I saw a queue of men standing obediently outside the double doors. Each was holding either a pink or blue teddy bear, a bag of grapes or a bunch of flowers in one hand, and a cigarette in the other. As the clock struck two, Sister Kelly opened the doors and welcomed them inside with the words: 'Come in, the lot of youse, but don't be lighting up any more o' them there cigarettes when those are finished. I don't want my ward contaminated.'

We followed the visitors, breathing in a lungful of smoke each. Margaret leaned into me and said conspiratorially, 'This bit is always touch and go.'

I had no idea what she meant until I caught sight of Sister Kelly throwing her arms up in the air. 'Oh, I'm sorry, I've done it again, haven't I?' she said as she pulled a stunned-looking young man back out through the curtains of bed thirteen. 'I do apologise, Mrs Charlesworth, so I do. Now then, Mr Clayton, your wife is just over here in the bed opposite. If you'll follow me ...'

'She does that all the time,' Margaret sniggered. 'Most of the women aren't bothered, but I don't suppose poor Mrs Charlesworth is very amused. She's suffering from engorged breasts and is strapped up with a couple of cot sheets holding up her bosom. No wonder Mr Clayton's eyes nearly popped out of his head!'

I clutched my sides laughing. It was fun as well as informative working on this ward, and I could tell I was going to enjoy my time here very much. It was very different to working at the MRI. For one thing it was less strict, but best of all the patients were well, and they were celebrating new life.

Chapter Ten

'Feeling the warmth of a baby's head in your hands, that new life, I'd honestly never experienced anything like it'

'Do you need a delivery, Linda?' Sister Houghton called.

'Oh yes, please!' I beamed, my heart giving a little skip.

'Follow me and scrub up quickly,' she instructed.

It was early March now and my official training as a pupil midwife had got off to a very busy start. I'd only been on Ward 19, the labour ward, for a matter of days, but I'd already been fortunate enough to step into the delivery rooms and witness a total of ten births. As Sister Houghton well knew, once a pupil midwife had witnessed ten births it was time for her to take part in a delivery herself, and to start ticking off her forty required deliveries.

By this time I'd also spent many hours attending lectures with three other pupil midwives, where we sweated over our *Textbook for Midwives* by Margaret F. Myles and fretted over how we would translate the hefty tome into reality when our big moment came and we actually got to take part in a delivery, instead of being mere observers. It was tantalisingly close. As we sat in those lectures we knew it would probably be just days before a new life would actually emerge into our very own hands, and now my moment was imminent.

The ten routine births I'd witnessed so far were very much like Mrs Hollingworth's, the first-ever delivery I'd seen at St

Mary's. I was grateful I'd had that valuable experience; it gave me a head start, I thought. I was also pleased that I already knew all about enemas and shaves, procedures with which I'd assisted on the female surgical ward at the MRI, as they were very much on the agenda here.

'The enema is performed to prevent a compacted bowel impeding the baby's journey down the birth canal,' Miss Greeves, one of our clinical instructors, explained during a lecture one day, 'while shaving is carried out to help reduce the risk of infection.'

Even though I knew this already I still looked on with interest as Miss Greeves stirred a mixture of soap and water in a jug and prepared a tube and funnel to demonstrate the process. In another lesson, much to my amazement, she instructed us in the art of making the perfect cup of tea, and I had learned to sit politely and always pay attention, regardless of how much I already knew about the subject.

'You must give an enema even if the patient has recently emptied her bowels, or even had diarrhoea,' Miss Greeves cautioned. 'It's a case of making sure the mixture is warm, inserting the tube up the lady's rectum and pouring the liquid through the tube, which is held high. This procedure is best done by two nurses working together.'

'Does anyone refuse?' a bold fellow student asked.

'No,' Miss Greeves replied, sounding rather surprised by the question. 'Not in my experience. Having an enema prior to delivery is always expected and accepted. The same goes for shaving.'

With that she sent us off to watch a friendly midwife called Barbara Lees shave a patient on the delivery ward. I looked on in alarm at the glinting blade on the razor Barbara was wielding, as it looked sharper than any I had encountered at the MRI.

'Don't look so afraid,' Barbara smiled. 'You'll be able to do this in your sleep before long. Sometimes we're shaving the woman in a mad panic just before the birth. You'll soon get used to it.'

I nodded uncertainly and felt glad the patient had her head turned away from us, as I'm sure I was wincing.

'So you're confident at giving enemas now?' Barbara asked, nodding towards Miss Greeves.

'Yes, I think so,' I replied, not wanting to distract Barbara from the job in hand.

'I don't suppose Miss Greeves told you this, but when it comes to enemas, all you need to remember is "high, hot and a hell of a lot!" That's what we always say here.'

Barbara laughed before lathering up some soap, applying it with cotton wool and setting to work with the razor. The unimpressed patient had lifted her nightgown under the raised sheets and now closed her eyes resignedly.

'One sister had me shaving a woman once who was literally pushing the baby out,' Barbara whispered. 'I was in such a panic, trying to holding the head in, that I cut the poor woman and actually made her bleed. I was terrified I'd left her vulnerable to infections instead of trying to prevent them!'

I enjoyed learning the ropes on the delivery ward, but what I really loved was watching babies being born.

I was absolutely thrilled each time I was called in to witness a birth with Sister Houghton, knowing I was getting closer to the moment when I would step forward and be a part of the magical process myself.

I'd seen Sister Houghton deliver three babies so far and it was a real education watching her work: hearing how she soothed and encouraged each woman as she waited for the baby's head to emerge and rotate, and seeing how she gently pulled the newborn down towards the bed. First the anterior shoulder appeared, then the posterior shoulder, before Sister Houghton hooked the baby under its armpits, heralding its thrilling arrival into the world.

During one of these deliveries, I hovered at the foot of the bed as Sister Houghton explained that this particular lady had started out breathing in gas and air from the large cylinder beside the bed to help her cope with the pain.

'When the gas and air didn't seem to help any more, I encouraged her to shout out,' Sister Houghton whispered. 'It often helps, but this lady started shouting out for more drugs. She's had an injection of the painkiller Pethilorfan, but of course that's nothing out of the ordinary.' Giving me a little wink, Sister Houghton added: 'You usually sense it's time to give it when they either start begging or swearing. Sometimes the women kick and bite too, I kid you not.'

I lapped up everything she said and did, feeling exhilarated at the spectacle of birth and wondering how incredible it would be to step into her shoes and actually help bring a baby into the world with my very own hands.

Now my moment had finally arrived. Had Sister Houghton really just said the words, 'Do you need a delivery, Linda?'? Yes, she had! I wasn't dreaming and the reality of the situation suddenly put me on red alert. Excited notions about the joy of being part of the miracle of birth started to slip away. Instead, I was overwhelmed with practical thoughts as words from my

Textbook for Midwives began to scramble through my head. 'Good wholesome cleanliness is the first prerequisite in midwifery …' it stated.

I followed Sister Houghton as she rushed into the delivery room. As quickly as possible, I attached a cloth mask over my nose and scrubbed my hands and arms up to my elbows using the soft brush on the sink. Next I put on a clean gown.

'Come on, Linda. Get your gloves on as fast as you can,' Sister Houghton urged. Her eyes flashed at me between her cap and mask. I couldn't see her lips but I could tell she was smiling. My heart was pounding as I pulled on my sterile gloves and joined Sister Houghton at the side of the bed.

'Look, we can already see baby's head,' she pointed.

I turned and saw that she was actually holding the slippery crown of the baby's head. In fact, she almost looked as though she was trying to push it back so the baby wasn't born before I got there. Excitement made my brain buzz, but something else was happening to me too. Little glass vials were being crunched up inside me, spilling cold liquid into my guts, making them contract. That's exactly what it felt like, and it was a feeling I hadn't experienced before in a delivery room. Responsibility was what filled those vials, I realised afterwards. I wasn't just a witness any more. I was dealing with the lives of two other human beings, and I could feel the weight of that responsibility pushing inside me as I reached out and let Sister Houghton replace her hands with mine.

'That's right,' she said softly as I touched the baby's head.

Adrenaline had taken over, flooding me, confusing me. Was I ecstatic or petrified? I wasn't sure if Sister Houghton was speaking to me or to the panting mother. For a split second, I was somewhere else. Touching the baby's head made everything fantastically real. Feeling the warmth of a baby's head in your hands, that new life, I'd honestly never experienced anything like it.

My hands were visibly shaking now and I could feel my gloves moving nervously over the baby's warm scalp. 'Now guard the perineum,' Sister Houghton said in a clear whisper. As she did so she placed her hands on top of mine, which immediately helped to still my trembling. She steered my right hand beneath the baby's head, so as to protect the mother's straining skin beneath and prevent it from tearing. I desperately didn't want the skin to tear. So far there had been no need for an episiotomy cut to help with this delivery and I didn't want anything at all to go wrong. I wanted this baby to be born absolutely perfectly.

'Now keep your fingers on the head ... steady, steady ...' Sister Houghton instructed quietly. In a louder voice she said efficiently: 'OK, just a little push please, Mrs Carmichael ... baby's head is nicely delivered.'

The crisp whisper was back in my ear a moment later. 'Check the cord isn't around the neck and wait for the external rotation of the head ... there we have it, baby's nicely on its side.' To the mother, she said loudly, 'Have you got another contraction for us?'

Mrs Carmichael did.

'OK now, Linda, you know what to do ... pull baby's head down and deliver the anterior shoulder ... lovely, lovely ... now sweep the posterior shoulder up and ...'

The baby plopped out beautifully onto the bed and my heart somersaulted. I was relieved and delighted to see it was a perfect little girl. With shaking hands, I lifted her carefully and looked at her in awe as she emitted her first little cry. I was the first person in the whole world to hold her. I felt so privileged, so delighted with myself. I'd taken on a huge responsibility and I'd carried it off. I'd delivered a baby!

I glanced at Mrs Carmichael's face. She was gazing at her baby and looked exhausted but blissfully content. I caught her eye for a moment and she gave me a wonderful, appreciative smile that made me glow even more.

I was so excited I could have turned a cartwheel across the delivery room floor, but I somehow managed to swallow my adrenaline rush and follow Sister Houghton's continual stream of steady, calm guidance.

As I clamped the cord and the little girl cried out once more, I wanted to cry too, but I kept myself in check. Once the placenta was successfully delivered a few minutes later, and as Sister Houghton cleaned and dressed and weighed the very beautiful black-haired baby, I had the honour of officially recording her birth in the hospital notes. I also had the pleasure of noting the details of the delivery in my own pupil midwife record book.

Using the fine fountain pen in my pocket, I wrote the mother's name, the sex of the baby, her seven pounds weight and the date and time of delivery as neatly as I possibly could, although my hands were still shaking with the thrill of it all. Sister Houghton signed the entry in my record book too, and I looked at it again and again, not quite believing what I was seeing and what I had done.

'I can deliver babies!' I thought. 'I've done it!' I was filled with an incredible feeling of achievement. Spontaneously, I gave Mrs Carmichael a hug and a kiss on the cheek.

'Thank you very much indeed!' I beamed.

'Thank you, Nurse!' she replied, looking a bit surprised.

'No, really, thank you. It couldn't have been a better birth,' I said, meaning every word, in every sense.

I'm not sure which of us was more flushed with pride, and in that moment I knew, without a shadow of a doubt, that I was going to absolutely love this job.

That evening Graham and I went for a drink and a meal at The Sportsman Inn with Colin and Marjorie, some neighbours we'd become friendly with. I enjoyed our evening out. The pub itself permanently smelled of smoke and, with its teak tables, low beams and heavy floral carpet, always felt a bit dark and dingy. It didn't bother me, though. The vast majority of my life revolved around either being at the hospital, shopping for food at Ashton Market or doing housework on my days off, then collapsing into bed tired out.

With Marjorie, I enjoyed switching off from work and chores and talking about other things. We often swapped make-up tips, all of which involved baby-blue eyeshadow, blue eyeliner and candyfloss-pink lipstick, and we giggled as we bought trousers with bottoms as wide as tents and skinny-rib polo-neck sweaters at Queenies on the market, where you had to go behind a flimsy curtain to try things on, risking flashing your underwear to other customers.

It was a Saturday night and I was very lucky to have the evening off, as pupil midwives were typically given the worst shifts. Graham complained about my rota from time to time, as we often had to turn down invitations because I was working, so I was pleased that for once my 'off duty' had been kind and I could celebrate a momentous day in my life with a night out with friends.

'To Linda, midwife extraordinaire,' Graham said, raising his glass of beer and giving my leg a squeeze under the table.

Marjorie and I chinked our glasses of Babycham and we all ordered scampi or chicken in a basket, which was a new fad at the pub and was all the rage.

'You've certainly had a more exciting day than I have,' Marjorie lamented. 'All I've delivered are the cashier reports for the manager at the bank.'

We laughed, and Graham began to tell our friends about our forthcoming trip to Torquay with his parents, which was a holiday we had planned for June, at the end of my Part One.

'Oh, you two have got it all worked out,' Marjorie said wistfully. 'I'll be slaving away behind the cash desk while you two are sunning yourselves. What a pair of lucky devils you are.'

I'd been so caught up in my training that I'd not taken stock of my life for a long while, though Marjorie's words rang true. Here I was, still aged just twenty-one, doing a responsible job I absolutely adored. Not only that, I was married to Graham and was lucky enough to be going on holiday to the south coast. Most people I knew only got as far as North Wales or perhaps Blackpool or the Lake District. Graham's business was growing very well, and we both had supportive families. He'd swapped his beloved bubble car for a black Austin he lovingly named Isobel, and we'd bought a glossy Red Setter called Sue, who we often took for walks around the lake at Stamford Park. Life was extremely good.

'Thanks for the compliment,' I said to Marjorie as I gave my husband a little hug. 'We're doing all right, aren't we, Graham?'

'You'll be having babies next, no doubt,' Marjorie teased.

'Not quite,' I said, hastily. 'I want to get my qualifications firmly out of the way first.'

My brother John and his wife Nevim had very recently announced they were expecting their first child in the autumn, which I was thrilled about. I still felt I had plenty of time before I needed to think about starting my own family. We'd have children together when it was right for both of us, and absolutely nothing could spoil our happiness.

A few days later I set off for work in unseasonably heavy snow. I didn't want to get my work shoes wet, so I put them in a bag that I wore diagonally across the back of my winter coat, and pulled on my favourite boots instead. Marjorie and I had recently bought a pair of kinky boots each from a fashionable little shoe shop in Stockport, and I adored them. Pulling the shiny black leather up to my knees and clicking my little heels either side of my Honda, I fancied myself as Diana Rigg in *The Avengers* as I ventured out into the crisp, white morning. The look wasn't quite right, of course, as the dress of my uniform was more maxi than mini, but nevertheless I felt good as I crossed the slushy streets of Ashton, the chorus of Nancy Sinatra's 'These Boots Were Made for Walking' whirling around my head as snowflakes collected on my helmet and gloves.

Turning right into Fountain Street and right again into the hospital grounds, I felt the wheels of the Honda slip a little. Cars couldn't drive up as close to the hospital as I could on my moped, so the snow on the path approaching the maternity unit at the back of the hospital grounds was still thick and fresh. I watched my front wheel kick up a flurry of powdery flakes, and thought what fun it was to be riding through the snow like this, free as a bird.

I felt the wheels slip again as I headed up past the entrance to Casualty, and without thinking I pulled hard on the throttle in an attempt to regain full control of the moped. This, of course, was a big mistake. In an instant, the bike seemed to take on a life of its own. My bag swung like a pendulum across my back, unbalancing me, and the whipping wheels of the moped accelerated with a roar. Seconds later I found myself being catapulted through the thick plastic swing doors leading into Casualty, where I landed, dazed and sore, in an undignified heap in front of the reception desk. I heard the moped crash to the ground behind me, and the smell of petrol fumes burned my nostrils.

'Are you all right, Nurse?' the stylish-looking receptionist said, dashing from behind her desk. 'Oh, dear, just look at your lovely go-go boots. What a shame.'

I sat up slowly and painfully, looked at my boots and wailed: 'I've only just bought them! And they cost me two pounds and ten shillings!'

One of my beloved kinky boots was ripped to pieces, my stockings were laddered and blood was oozing from a large gash down the side of my right calf, which began to sting sharply.

A male Casualty nurse rushed over to help me up and dispatched a colleague to remove the moped, which I noticed had left a nasty black skid mark across the thick grey lino. Hopping gingerly into a side bay, I glanced around and saw an audience of bemused and somewhat amused faces staring back at me from the waiting area. What an unexpected spectacle they had witnessed, and what a sight I must have looked in my nurse's uniform and shredded boots.

'Let's get those boots off first,' the male nurse said, suppressing a smile. 'I'm afraid you won't be "go-going" anywhere else in those!'

I laughed reluctantly at his silly pun, but my pride was nursing a large bruise, which throbbed in time with my pulse as I lay on a couch and suffered the embarrassment of having to remove my tattered stockings while the now highly amused male nurse prepared to stitch the cut in my leg.

'How did you lose your way?' he asked, straight-faced, as he set to work putting five stitches in my wound. 'Was the path outside a bit kinky?'

He laughed at his own joke while I managed to smile gamely. I think it was either that or I might have wailed again. 'I'm not going to be allowed to forget this in a hurry, am I?' I said resignedly.

'Probably not!' came the perky reply. 'It's not every day a pupil midwife comes crashing into Casualty in such dramatic style. Look on the bright side; at least you were in the right place to get yourself patched up, eh?'

When I stepped tentatively through the doors of the delivery ward later that morning I was greeted by Barbara Lees, who asked me if I was up to observing a Caesarean after my 'incident'. Word had clearly spread like wildfire, and I suspected I was something of a laughing stock. Despite still being in considerable pain I was keen to minimise my embarrassment, and I readily agreed to accompany Barbara to theatre.

'Come on then, you'll have to be quick,' she beckoned.

I had witnessed two routine Caesareans already, and a mental image of them pinned itself to the front of my brain. The drill was the same both times, and I pictured myself wheeling the patient downstairs to the hospital theatre, putting on my mask and scrubbing up meticulously, letting the water run away from my hands right up to my elbows, drying my hands on the sterile towel and asking a colleague to tie me into my gown as I pulled on each glove, making sure not to touch the outsides of them.

The woman would be on the table, already anaesthetised. Women always had a general anaesthetic for Caesarean sections as spinal anaesthetics, or epidurals, would not be used for many years to come.

Today, everything appeared as I expected when I entered the theatre with Barbara. The patient, Audrey Wainwright, was draped in green towels, one of which had a window cut out revealing her abdomen. Barbara told me that Mrs Wainwright had been quite poorly with high blood pressure, which was what had prompted the Caesarean.

'Doctor thought it best not to risk it getting any higher,' Barbara explained. 'She's almost full term, so it wasn't worth taking the risk of things going wrong at this late stage.'

High blood pressure, I knew, could threaten the life of both mother and baby, and was to be avoided at all costs. I was very glad Mrs Wainwright was in safe hands, having her baby delivered sensibly early.

I could see by the way the surgeon had draped the theatre towels around her abdomen that Mrs Wainwright was destined to have a horizontal incision, known as a bikini cut, rather than a larger classical cut, which would run vertically down from the navel. This, I knew, would only have been used if the baby was very distressed, and I felt reassured that this was therefore not an emergency situation.

I stood near the operating table, concentrating hard and watching very carefully as the surgeon got to work. He cut the skin and cauterised the bleeding with a hot diathermy needle, then with remarkably impressive speed he began cutting through the layers of muscle and fat to get through to the uterus.

I watched in fascination, mesmerised by the flashing steel and the surgeon's nimble, busy hands, which were flooded in brightness from the theatre lights overhead. Any minute now the surgeon would pierce the membranes, I anticipated. The baby was tantalisingly close to being born. In my peripheral vision I was aware of the scrub nurse laying out a clean scalpel, as well as dissecting forceps and curved scissors on a table beside the bed. I saw her pass a swab to the surgeon, who mopped the wound. Now I saw a suction nozzle, too, in readiness for the moment the foetal sac would be punctured, which I predicted would be any second now. In my mind's eye I was following the pages in my midwifery textbook, as well as remembering the two Caesareans I'd seen before. I knew what came next and was almost seeing each move a split second before it happened.

Suddenly, I became aware of the surgeon muttering something about blood pressure. The mother's blood pressure was high, too high. I had not anticipated this turn of events, or the uncharacteristically sharp edge to the surgeon's naturally soft voice. I felt my nerves tense as I tore my eyes from the open abdomen and swept them around the theatre table. To my horror, I saw the surgeon and Barbara catch eyes and share an anxious glance. The surgeon broke the waters expertly, and seconds later he was lifting the baby out, holding the little body upside down. This was to facilitate pulmonary drainage. I knew that's what the textbook said, but I sensed this was not a textbook birth.

I instinctively took a step back. My textbook was being torn up in my head. Barbara glanced at the clock, noting the time of birth. The surgeon was using clamps and scissors to cut the cord. I braced myself for the silence, sensing that we were not going to hear this baby cry. I could see that it wasn't moving, but that can happen. That's what I was thinking, desperately.

Barbara wrapped the baby in a sterile cotton blanket. First she used mechanical suction to clear his airway. Done. Good – there was mucus and the blockage was gone. Now oxygen to resuscitate him, fast. That's what he needed urgently.

'Get the paediatrician!' Barbara shouted. The baby's skin was white, not pink. He looked limp, fast asleep. His cord, which had been clamped and tied, looked feeble and floppy.

Barbara extended his head slightly, lifting his chin up, as she placed him in the resuscitaire and set to work, trying to revive him under the heat and light, with oxygen pumped through a tiny nozzle. She also gave him cardiac massage, gently pushing his chest with two fingers in quick succession, time and time again.

'Yes, that's right,' she was saying earnestly, almost pleadingly. 'Yes, keep going. Keep going, go on. Please breathe.'

The paediatrician ran in and tried for many minutes to revive the baby, but the little boy remained still and never took a breath. He had needed more oxygen in the womb, and now he was beyond help. Tragically, this baby had been born just too late, and we had no chance of saving him. He was stillborn.

The realisation hit me very hard, almost like a physical blow to my body. The muscles around my heart tightened and I felt choked and helpless as I stood in shocked silence, watching the paediatrician shake his head sadly and step away from the resuscitaire, head bowed.

Barbara wrapped the baby up extra-carefully and laid him tenderly in a prepared cot. He looked perfect, just fast asleep. I started to cry, and I could see that Barbara was close to tears too.

'She will be waking up soon,' Barbara whispered in a thin, quivering voice.

I sniffed back my tears, thinking Barbara was cautioning me not to cry in front of the bereaved mother. In fact, as she continued to talk I realised Barbara was simply letting me know what would happen next.

'I will take the baby away before she wakes,' she explained.

Her words highlighted the finality of it all. The baby was dead, and that was the right thing to do. I knew that. We'd discussed it in class one day. The tutor had told us clearly: 'The appropriate action is to remove the baby before the mother sees it, with the minimum of fuss. It is too distressing for a woman to have to see her dead baby. It is best to wait for her to ask questions and let the truth dawn on her. If this task falls to you, tell the truth and offer condolence, but choose your words carefully. For example, you must never tell her it will be all right next time, because you do not know that.'

I remembered that lesson vividly, because it had jolted me rudely back to my time on Casualty, when the young car crash victim, Tabitha, had died. I had already made the dreadful error of telling a mother things would be all right when they wouldn't be, and I knew I would never, ever repeat that mistake.

As Barbara wheeled the baby out of the hushed theatre in his cot, unwelcome images entered my head. I knew that babies like this were sometimes placed discreetly inside another person's coffin, so as to give them a dignified burial without putting the parents through the ordeal of a funeral. I didn't want to think about this, but in my shock I couldn't control my thoughts. It was practically unheard of back then to hold a funeral for a stillborn baby. I couldn't bear to think of this little mite being laid beside a stranger, or even left alone in the mortuary. Whatever happened, it was certainly not what his mum had planned, and I felt utterly devastated.

Mercifully, Barbara had returned by the time Mrs Wainwright began to stir. I hadn't met the lady before this day, and despite my training I didn't have a clue what to say or do. Barbara stroked the back of her hand as her eyes flickered and she slowly became aware of her surroundings.

'What is it?' Mrs Wainwright asked, disorientated. 'Wh-what's happened?'

'I'm terribly sorry …' Barbara started, which made Mrs Wainwright snap her eyes wide open and look down at her deflated belly. She had been stitched by now, and a large sterile pad lay across her empty abdomen.

'Wh-wh-where's my baby?' she asked, panic rising in her voice.

'I'm afraid your baby didn't live,' Barbara said compassionately. She tilted her head to one side and leaned over Mrs Wainwright. For a moment I wondered if she was going to give the poor woman a hug, but then I realised Barbara was positioned in such a way as to stop Mrs Wainwright from falling should she try to get up off the bed.

'You had a little boy but he didn't take a breath. I'm so very sorry.'

I took hold of Mrs Wainwright's other hand and held it tight as her tears started to flow uncontrollably.

'What will I tell my Gordon?' she wailed. 'What will I tell 'im? We wanted this baby so much! Why did he have to die? Why didn't he take a breath? We wanted him so much. Did you know, we tried for years and years to have this baby? Years and years!'

Each word she spoke sounded more urgent, more desperate than the last.

'Why?' she shouted eventually. 'What was wrong with him? TELL ME, TELL ME, TELL ME NOWWWWW!'

Barbara caught my eye and gave a little shake of her head. I knew not to try to answer. She had suffered from dangerously high blood pressure in the latter stages of her pregnancy and, as far as we knew, that is what had led to this calamitous outcome. A doctor would explain more in due course. It wasn't our place to discuss that with her, and it certainly wasn't the time.

'The doctor will come and see you soon,' Barbara began to explain, but Mrs Wainwright wasn't listening. She threw our hands away with an unexpected amount of force and let out a series of howls that came from somewhere very dark and deep within her wounded belly. I didn't know that bereavement had a sound until that moment, and I had never heard anything so distressing. Each wretched wail ripped up from her belly, spilling unimaginable pain into the air I breathed.

'In that theatre, it really dawned on me how precious life is,' I said to Graham that night.

He'd already let me have a good cry, and now he was letting me talk.

'I mean, we all know life is precious, but I don't think I realised just *how* precious life is, until today. I can't get over what happened, I really can't. That baby should have lived. It had survived for months and months and was just waiting to be born. Why didn't we deliver Mrs Wainwright earlier? Why didn't the doctors realise he was going to die if we waited until today? It's just not fair. That's what I can't accept. Some girls have sex once behind the bike shed and end up with babies they don't even want. Others have babies to order, and to them it's like shelling peas. Then you get someone like poor Mrs Wainwright. Her baby was longed for. She and her husband had been trying for years to have a baby. They wanted him so much, and yet it has ended in the most terrible tragedy. It's so unfair. You should have heard her, Graham, she was absolutely hysterical.'

Graham just held me tight, which is exactly what I wanted. 'Tomorrow's another day, love,' he said. 'I know it's hard, but it's a part of your job. I know you can do it. Tomorrow will be better, you'll see.'

I slept very badly, and each time I closed my eyes I saw the poor dead baby's peaceful, motionless face. Eventually, I sat bolt upright in bed. A shard of early morning sunlight dazzled me through a knife-thin gap in the bedroom curtains. I blinked my eyes tight shut and everything went blood red, which terrified me for a moment. Then I realised, to my great relief, that this was simply my own blood I could see inside my sunlit eyelids. Silly Linda. Silly, silly Linda. Everything is OK. Get up now, Linda, you've got work to do.

Once I was fully awake and putting on my uniform, I reasoned with myself. It was perfectly natural to be upset about that poor little soul, of course it was. I wouldn't be human if I didn't get upset. Dealing with tragedies like that was part of life, and part of my job. If you are going to work at the sharp end of bringing new life into the world, you have to be strong enough to cope when things go wrong. 'I can do it,' I told myself. 'Sometimes it's going to be tough, Linda, but Graham is right. You are in the right job. You must be the best midwife you possibly can be.'

Despite my reasoning, I knew the feelings of devastation at losing that baby would never fully leave me, and I was right. Even to this day, every last detail of that birth is etched on my memory, and I can still feel the pain of the loss.

My heart sank when the delivery bell rang out on the ward later that morning. Normally I sprang to attention, running to sister to ask if I could attend, clutching my record book expectantly, hoping I would be able to tick off another one of my forty deliveries.

Today was different, though. Despite Graham's support, and the pep talk I'd given myself that morning, I couldn't get away from the fact I was still very upset about Mrs Wainwright. Devastated, in fact. Her delivery pushed me closer to completing my target of six Caesarean sections, but I hadn't felt a jot of triumph when Sister Houghton signed the relevant page in my record book.

Reluctantly, I entered the delivery room after Sister Houghton had come to find me and chivvy me along.

'It's a first baby, all routine,' she said with a sunny smile. 'Come along, chop, chop! Baby won't wait for you, Linda!'

I tried to be positive and think about my wonderful first delivery with Mrs Carmichael, and I prayed to God this next one would run as smoothly as hers.

I felt a whoosh of hot air fill my mask as I stepped up close to the bed. I'd been so tense I'd been holding my breath, but I hadn't realised it until that moment. An experienced midwife called Val was telling the sweating mother to pant and not to push, even if she felt the urge. I could just see the top of the baby's scalp.

'I'm going to do an episiotomy,' Val announced, and I watched as she injected local anaesthetic swiftly into the perineum, in between contractions. The labouring mother did not appear to have been consulted about this procedure, though she did not object. From the midwife's point of view it was a disgrace to have a tear. It was deemed far better to have a clean surgical cut than risk a ragged laceration, and women having their first baby seemed willing to accept that the midwife might make this cut routinely to 'widen the vulval orifice', as the textbook described it.

'I'm just going to make a little cut to help baby on its way,' Val explained to this mother in a matter-of-fact tone. She waited until the next contraction came so the skin was taut and stretched before making one precise incision just over an inch long in the woman's flesh. With a swift wipe of a gauze swab, the bleeding was gone and another inch of the baby's scalp was revealed.

Val let me take over as soon as the episiotomy was completed, and it turned out to be another perfect birth. There was only one difference from Mrs Carmichael's delivery. I still got an unbelievable rush of excitement when I felt the new life in my hands, but this time my hands weren't trembling quite as much as they had the first time. I think I'd been too intrigued by the spectacle of the episiotomy to think about my nerves, and I astonished myself by talking calmly to the labouring mother as I copied Sister Houghton's soothing phrases before announcing confidently and triumphantly: 'Well done! It's a girl!'

That's how I got my second delivery, and it raised my spirits no end. I was buzzing all over again, and I couldn't wait to deliver my next thirty-eight babies, and more! In fact, in that moment I wanted to deliver hundreds and hundreds of babies, if not thousands! That was my youthful dream and, as ambitious as it seemed, I really wished it would come true.

Chapter Eleven

'Knickers and tights off, ladies!'

'Linda, forceps delivery!' Barbara Lees bellowed above the sound of the trilling bell that announced a delivery was imminent. 'Put those bunnies down and come quick!'

'Bunnies' was the name we gave to the big thick sanitary towels dished out to the women after they gave birth. They were useful for all sorts of other things, and I'd often seen midwives soothing a patient's brow with a bunny that had been soaked in cold water, or using one as a sponge to mop up a spillage.

I had been about to neatly re-stock the store cupboard and was fondly remembering the time one very posh lady had complained to a colleague: 'Nurse! I do hope you are not wiping my brow with a sanitary towel!'

When the midwife admitted that she was in fact using a bunny as a facecloth the well-spoken lady suddenly decided that it felt so refreshing on her warm forehead that she didn't mind after all, which made us all smile.

Barbara's urgent cry snapped me out of my daydream and I threw the bunnies in a haphazard heap before chasing after her. Dr Franklin had given a detailed lecture about forceps deliveries, and I was intrigued to see how his vivid descriptions and explanations would come to life in the delivery room.

To tell the truth, I was a little fearful too, as the collection of forceps he had displayed in the school room looked more like instruments of torture than surgical instruments. The Kielland forceps were frighteningly big, while Neville-Barnes and Simpson's forceps were smaller yet, I imagined, could be just as brutal.

'Kielland forceps are only to be used by the very skilled consultant or registrar,' Dr Franklin had cautioned solemnly. 'It is not within the midwife's province to decide when forceps should be applied, but she must be aware of the various indications for their use.'

He went on to list a multitude of complications that may necessitate a forceps delivery, including maternal or foetal distress or high blood pressure. 'When it's not appropriate to perform a Caesarean section, forceps should be called for,' he explained. Suction using a ventouse vacuum extractor attached to the scalp was another option at this junction, Dr Franklin added, but this was not as commonly used.

The type of forceps chosen depended on the problem encountered. Before the use of forceps, the mother would always require an episiotomy and a 'pudendal nerve block', which was an injection delivered into the perineum to anaesthetise the nerves supplying the pelvic floor, vagina and vulva. Her legs would be put in lithotomy, meaning her feet would be raised above hip level and placed in stirrups, to give the doctor the best possible access to the baby.

As if this wasn't alarming enough, Dr Franklin had not finished yet. 'The aim is to put the forceps around the baby's ears and pull at the same time as the labouring mother is pushing. Sometimes the baby is born with large red marks on its face, and sometimes a baby delivered this way may be a little irritable, or can be shocked. It is not uncommon for the baby to have a high-pitched cry, which is a result of the traumatic nature of the birth. A difficult forceps delivery can leave a baby severely traumatised, though this is, of course, extremely uncommon.'

I had come to respect Dr Franklin, despite his reputation for being rude and insulting to young girls who fell pregnant by accident. There weren't many of those, thank goodness. I had only heard tales of two or three teenage pregnancies in my first four months here, and had not actually encountered one myself. The last outburst I'd overheard from Dr Franklin, however, had been just days earlier, when I heard him berating an overweight young girl.

'Just look at you!' he scoffed angrily. 'What a big fat thing you are! Not only do you need to stop having intercourse out of wedlock, you need to stop being such a greedy girl!'

He was outrageous, but from what I overheard the girl took it on the chin and spluttered that she was really sorry.

Despite his faults, I enjoyed having lectures with Dr Franklin. He was surprisingly patient with us pupil midwives and always endeavoured to answer our questions at length. He would discuss deliveries we'd been a part of in minute detail and share his knowledge generously, albeit sometimes very graphically. This meant that when I eventually did see my first forceps birth, I felt very well prepared and imagined I knew it all.

However, I stopped in my tracks as I entered the delivery room hot on Barbara's heels that day. The mother was screaming relentlessly. I'd never heard such an ear-splitting wail. If I didn't know better, I'd have though she was being brutally attacked. My heart went out to her, and I watched and listened in stunned, horrified silence.

Dr Franklin was shouting at the midwife, telling her brusquely to 'Get the patient pushing, will you?' while he wielded the dreaded Kielland forceps, grunting and heaving and sweating as he struggled to pull the baby out.

'Aaaarrrghhh!' the woman screeched. 'It's killing me! Make it stop!'

'Push now!' the midwife implored. I could see the woman's red sore heels grinding into the stirrups as she raged against her pain. The gas and air she had been given, and the Pethidine, were clearly not helping enough. It was as if she were rigged up to a medieval torture bed, as her legs were strapped firmly down and her hands were desperately clawing the air.

The traumatic din and strenuous pushing and pulling persisted for a full ten minutes before the red-faced baby was literally dragged out into the world. He let out an incredibly high-pitched cry, which I realised was about the only thing about the procedure I'd been prepared for after all.

I watched anxiously, sweat pricking my brow, as Dr Franklin delivered the placenta before suturing the perineum. The process took quite some time because the patient needed a great deal of stitches. I winced in sympathy each time the needle went in, but when I stole a look at the mother's face, to my surprise and relief she was smiling radiantly.

'I'm going to call him Henry,' she said sweetly, gazing at her baby adoringly as he was cleaned and weighed and put in a nappy. 'After Henry Cooper,' she chuckled. 'Little bruiser!'

A few weeks later I sat in the ward kitchen eating a ginger biscuit, drinking a cup of tea and giving my throbbing feet a well-earned rest after a round of temperature and blood pressure checks. It was May now, and I was well on the way to completing Part One.

At the end of June, Graham and I were heading off to Torquay for our week in the sun with his parents before I would begin Part Two in July, spending four months out in the district with community midwife Mrs Tattersall.

I flicked through my record book and felt very satisfied to see that I had managed to fulfil my obligation to witness six Caesareans, six forceps deliveries (of which the subsequent five were markedly less dramatic than the first), and five out of my six required breech births. I had not expected it to be so easy to tick these complicated births off my list in a matter of a few weeks, but the hospital was so busy I could easily have witnessed many more.

There was an old copy of the *Manchester Evening News* lying on the counter top, and I snatched a few moments to read a report about The Beatles' break-up. Tragically, Paul McCartney had announced that they were to disband on the day he released his first solo album, and I was dismayed to read about fall-outs between the Fab Four, and how the others had asked Paul to wait until the last Beatles album, *Let It Be*, came out, before releasing his own. I loved every record The Beatles had released, and I hummed one of my favourites, 'Love Me Do', as I read the latest news, feeling heartbroken.

'Nurse Buckley, what are you doing?'

I was startled to see none other than Miss Sefton looming in the kitchen doorway, hands on hips.

I opened my mouth to speak but she answered the question herself with the words: 'I know you! Eating ginger biscuits no less! I can smell them on your breath!'

'I'm very sorry ...' I stuttered, knowing that she hated to see any of her staff eating on duty, even in the privacy of the ward kitchen. Simply sipping a cup of tea during a shift was unacceptable in her book, and she expected her staff only to take refreshments during official break times, which this was not.

'Apology accepted,' she sighed, sounding calmer, 'but don't let this happen again. Now then, Nurse Buckley, how are you getting on with your deliveries?'

Peering at my open record book, Miss Sefton's eyes fell on my tally of five breech births – the only section that had not been signed off as completed in my Part One.

'I see you have another breech to witness,' she said, raising her eyebrows. 'I know it is not always the easiest target to reach, and of course we would not wish for more breech births, ordinarily.'

Usually it was possible to tell if the baby was breech by palpating the abdomen, but, with only the aid of their hands to feel the shape of the baby, midwives and doctors occasionally got it wrong. Either way, it didn't affect the delivery plans. Women expecting to have a breech birth generally had to battle bravely on with a vaginal delivery. Back then everyone knew you only got a Caesarean if a vaginal birth was absolutely out of the question, and the mother's or the baby's life was in danger. The prospect of heightened anxiety and trauma during a breech delivery was not a good enough reason to go under the knife in those days, not by a long way.

I'd found each breech birth nerve-racking to watch, seeing a little foot or bottom appear first instead of the top of the head. The women sometimes suffered from dreadful stress, and during each birth the tension in the delivery room ran so high it was practically tangible.

'It may have been fortunate for you that I caught you here today,' Miss Sefton announced. 'If I am not mistaken, I believe Dr Franklin has a breech birth imminent. You may be wise to put away the ginger biscuits and seek him out.'

I did as I was told with mixed feelings. I desperately wanted to tick off my sixth and final observation of a breech delivery, but I felt quite sick with nerves that day. The atmosphere in the delivery room would be highly charged, and I knew I would spend the entire birth feeling desperately sorry for the labouring mother, and fearing for the life of the baby as it made its clumsy entrance into the world.

In the early stages the mother would be crying and shouting for more drugs, complaining that the pain-relieving gas and air or injection of Pethilorfan were no use at all, and the midwife would be trying to keep her as calm as possible.

I found Dr Franklin in Room 4. The staff midwife, Val, informed me that the delivery was going quite well and the baby was already halfway out. I knew that a calm atmosphere was of paramount importance at this stage, but an almost unnatural quiet filled the entire delivery room. I would have preferred hollering and cursing to this eerie silence, and I felt instantly afraid for the safety of the baby.

Dr Franklin acknowledged my presence with a brief nod as I tiptoed up beside him. He was seated at the foot of the bed, between the woman's legs. I could see this was a 'footling' breech delivery, also known as an 'extended breech' delivery, meaning the baby was arriving legs first rather than bottom first.

To my surprise I recognised the mother as a customer from my parents' bakery. Her name was Philippa Frodsham and I had served her occasionally when I helped out behind the counter as a teenager. She seemed terribly snobbish and was 'partial to parkin', I recalled, which was one of my father's speciality cakes. Her husband was either a dentist or a chiropodist, I couldn't remember which.

I was accustomed to seeing Philippa buttoned into expensive, richly coloured smock coats with matching hats, twittering on about meeting the ladies for lunch or discussing private schooling with other well-heeled customers. Now, the only clue to her social status was the glamorous red satin Alice band still clamped firmly across her neatly bobbed blonde hair.

I caught her eye and smiled, and she gave me a soft smile back. I had no idea whether she recognised me or was just grateful to see another friendly female face in the room. That said, it always amazed me that ladies like Philippa, who were normally refined and even prudish, were never coy about having a man deliver their baby.

Husbands were banished to the corridors during internal examinations, let alone births, but it was perfectly acceptable for a male doctor to be at the 'business end' of a delivery. Male doctors were revered, in fact, and were especially glorified if they were consultants. Time and time again I saw patients looking up to the senior male doctors almost as if they were gods. I had to admit that there were times when their skills earned them that privilege, however, and this was certainly one of those occasions.

I saw that one little foot and leg were already dangling, and Dr Franklin was in the process of gently teasing the second leg down, his hand inside the vagina as he unfolded the limb and hooked it free, ever so slowly and carefully. With two legs cleanly delivered, Val fetched a sterile blanket and Dr Franklin wrapped the little boy's legs together to keep them warm, and so he could get a better grip on the baby.

Blood seeped onto the white blanket, patching it with red. I could see that Mrs Frodsham had had an episiotomy. Normally the pressure of the head on the cut skin stemmed the bleeding, but of course in this case the head was coming out last, which made the slack wound ooze blood.

An injection of the local anaesthetic Lignocaine had been administered and Mrs Frodsham did not appear to be in any great pain, but I saw that her usually smooth, unruffled face was creased with anxiety and had a sheen of perspiration. Val soothed her brow with a cool flannel, reassuring her ever so quietly that she was doing extremely well. 'It's very important that you stay calm,' Val whispered. 'We need you to stay calm for the baby.'

I knew that if the baby was delivered too rapidly at this stage his fragile little head could be damaged. Also, with him half in and half out, we didn't want him to get over-stimulated and try to take a breath before his head was safely delivered. I watched intently as Dr Franklin expertly teased the two little arms down from above the baby's head, a process that took three long minutes. Seeing ten little fingers and two little arms descend was absolutely wonderful, but I was still tight with nerves. Dr Franklin proceeded to deliver the shoulders with what looked like incredible ease, though I knew this was a manoeuvre that was extremely tricky and fraught with difficulty. I was watching a master at work, and it was something else to behold.

Dr Franklin now rose to his feet, so as to prepare to deliver the head safely. As the nape of the baby's neck was now visible, on the next contraction Dr Franklin grasped his ankles gently and, with slight traction, carried his body up over the mother's abdomen. Mrs Frodsham looked on nervously but silently.

Her baby's legs were now in her line of vision even though the delivery was not complete yet. She was doing very well indeed, and was breathing steadily.

I actually held my breath when the next contraction arrived, watching as Dr Franklin skilfully delivered the baby's head as gradually as could be. He didn't call for forceps; there was no need. I let out my breath with tremendous relief.

I could see the baby's face at last. His little nose and mouth were free now, and I watched with delight as he took his first breath. I silently thanked God that the delivery was completed with textbook precision, and I had tears in my eyes as I saw Mrs Frodsham's anxious face finally relax into a broad, incredulous smile. The relief when she finally saw her son's scrunched-up little face was an absolute joy to witness. I would seek her out on the postnatal ward in a day or two and take her some of my father's finest parkin, I thought giddily. That was the least she deserved.

When I left the delivery room that day, I noticed that Dr Franklin had watery eyes too, and I remembered Margaret Mulligan's words on my very first day here. 'Don't worry about Dr Franklin,' she had said. 'He's got a soft heart underneath all the bluster.' Now I had finally seen it, and I admired him all the more for it.

To complete Part One of my course, I also worked in the Special Care Baby Unit (SCBU) and in the antenatal clinic. I didn't feel at all comfortable in Special Care, and was very relieved that I was simply required to observe the tiny babies in their incubators. All babies below five pounds in weight had to be taken to Special Care, where they were looked after by specially trained nurses.

It was very hot and very regimented in Special Care. Babies were fed every one to three hours, and I had to help make up the feeds. To prevent the spread of infection nurses wore a different gown over their uniforms to attend to each baby. Only very few babies were well enough to be fed by their mothers.

I learned that a diabetic mother's baby could be big but immature, which accounted for one or two of the larger babies I saw. However, the majority were so fragile they didn't look like babies at all, and that was distressing to see. They appeared very pink, with shiny skin. Some looked like the skinned rabbits my mum used to make rabbit pie with, which was an image that upset me but wouldn't leave me. I hated to see babies like that, attached to tubes and machines to help their tiny lungs inflate. Survival rates were low in those days, and I couldn't look at the babies without fearing desperately for their perilously premature lives. It was like being suspended in a strange, dangerous world, where life and death played a heart-stopping game of chase. I couldn't wait for my time there to end.

The antenatal clinic, by contrast, was a breath of fresh air. I loved seeing the women waddling in, full of optimism. The clinic was in a draughty, hut-like unit separated from the main hospital building. It was barely big enough to swing a cat in and it always seemed madly busy, but I loved its vibe.

Women who were pregnant with their first babies would attend every two weeks for a routine urine test and blood pressure check, and sometimes for internal examinations too. Those who already had children didn't attend the clinic so often, as they would also be seen at home by a community midwife.

The midwife would weigh each patient, measure the woman's stomach using her hands, and listen to the baby's heartbeat using a Pinard stethoscope, which is like a little trumpet. A doctor or consultant would also perform a brief examination of the abdomen and record observations, and they'd do an internal examination if required.

In lectures we'd been told that this part of the midwife's job was as much about talking, listening and observing as it was about the practicalities of routine tests and examinations. I found it a pleasure to share in each woman's excitement, and I embraced the challenge of recognising when all was not well, whether it be swelling that might signal the onset of pre-eclampsia, or a personal problem the woman needed to get off her chest. Preventing trouble was much more satisfying than dealing with the after-effects of misfortune or calamity, which is how I saw Special Care. I felt useful and very much at home in the antenatal clinic.

'Knickers and tights off, ladies!' Sister Baxter called to a row of waiting women on my first morning.

I giggled as I watched them obediently take turns to go inside the cubicles and remove their undergarments before entering the examination room. This preparation was done so as not to waste valuable time with the doctor.

I enjoyed watching the easy camaraderie amongst the women waiting to be seen.

'Took me half an hour to get me tights on this mornin',' one lady griped when it was her turn in the cubicle. Complaining that she had struggled to reach her toes she remarked, 'I'd have been better off coming in with bare legs!'

'I know,' another chipped in. 'Ooooh-er! Wait up!' she added suddenly. 'There's a man over there!'

Each waiting woman turned her head to the open door at the end of the corridor, where a shy-looking young man was hovering nervously.

Sister Baxter was nose to nose with him in a flash. 'What do you want? You can wait outside!' she ordered bossily, taking hold of his arm and practically pushing him out the door.

'Honestly!' Sister Baxter huffed, turning to address the gaping ladies, who were all tut-tutting. 'I do apologise for that. What *was* he thinking?'

None of the ladies owned up to knowing the errant father-to-be, but his exit prompted a lively discussion about the ridiculous things men did when their wives were pregnant.

'My old man asked if he could go to an away match in Blackburn on the weekend the baby's due. Told me: "Don't worry, I'll make sure I get to a phone box at half time." Cheeky beggar!'

'I'd be grateful if I were you,' another piped up. 'Mine asked me if he was allowed to come in the delivery room and watch the birth!'

Everybody fell about laughing, especially a couple of middle-aged women who were accompanying their pregnant daughters.

'The idea of it!' one of the older women scoffed. 'Can you imagine? Your father would have fainted on the spot if he'd seen me giving birth to you. What a carry-on that would have been! As if women haven't got enough to cope with without husbands adding to their woes ...'

I chuckled as I left the clinic that sunny afternoon at the end of June. That was my last shift before my holiday in Torquay but, much more importantly, it was my last shift of Part One, which Miss Sefton informed me I had now completed 'competently'.

'You show great promise, Nurse Buckley,' she told me before I left. 'I imagine you will do very well in the community.'

I was thrilled to bits. After my experience in the antenatal clinic, I was really looking forward to venturing out into the district. I imagined it would be a great privilege to get to know the pregnant mums more personally before they gave birth, and to be a part of their whole adventure.

Graham's parents, Edith and Bill, had organised our holiday and had booked us into a pretty chalet called 'The Haven' near the beach. Graham drove us down to the south coast in 'Isobel', which he had specially polished for the occasion. His father sat in the front and navigated while my mother-in-law and I shared the back seat. I wore a new cream silk blouse, grey tight-fitting trousers with bell bottoms and some fashionable black wedge heels. Graham had bought me a Siamese silver ring as a 'well done' present for passing Part One, which I wore proudly on my finger. I was delighted that I'd be able to wear it for the whole week without taking it on and off as I had to do for work every day.

It took twelve hours to reach our destination, and this gave Edith and me ample time to chat.

'I'm so proud of you, Linda,' she beamed affectionately. 'Being a midwife is such a wonderful career. My Graham is very lucky to have found a lovely wife like you.'

She asked me lots of questions about hospital life, delivering babies and how I felt about the inevitable tragedies that rubbed alongside the joys of childbirth. I enjoyed the chance to chat, especially with someone as genuinely interested and inquisitive as my mother-in-law.

'What doesn't kill you makes you stronger,' I heard myself saying to Edith at one point, and I remembered first hearing it in the MRI when I was a wet-behind-the-ears eighteen-year-old. It had been one of Miss Morgan's stoical mantras, which was often regurgitated by her sisters. 'Listen to me,' I thought to myself. 'Only twenty-two and churning out those words of experience!'

Edith was very good company and it felt as if we talked about everything under the sun as we lamented the lack of motorways and navigated the network of twisting A and B roads leading to Torquay. It was particularly refreshing to chat about the big wide world outside Ashton General, which I rarely got the time to do.

'What will it mean for the NHS with the Conservatives now in power?' Edith asked keenly at one point.

I didn't really have a clue, but I'd heard good things about Edward Heath, our brand new Prime Minister. I thought he could be quite good for the country, though I wasn't political at all and my rather vague view was based on hearsay.

The compensation that had finally been agreed for Thalidomide victims was another topic raised. I didn't know the details but I welcomed news of the long-awaited settlement wholeheartedly. The morning sickness drug that caused such devastating birth defects had been withdrawn several years before I began training as a nurse, let alone a midwife, but just hearing the word 'Thalidomide' made me sad. I could vividly imagine the trauma of delivering a baby with stunted limbs, and was very glad I had never had to do anything like that, though I knew some of my older colleagues had. The aftershocks were still reverberating around midwifery circles, and it was only ever talked about in hushed, regretful tones.

'What do you think about Paul McCartney leaving The Beatles?' Edith asked next, to my relief. This was a subject I was happy to talk about.

'I'm absolutely gutted! I bought *Let It Be* the other week, and I just can't believe it's their last album. I only hope John Lennon will have a solo career too if the Beatles don't sort their differences out. Do you think he will?'

'I'm sure he will, Linda,' came the reply, which was exactly what I wanted to hear. We had a little sing-song after that, thinking we were so witty singing 'The Long and Winding Road' as we wended our way slowly southwards.

The four of us spent our days in Torquay sunbathing on towels and deckchairs on the beach, and each night Graham's dad treated us all to a slap-up dinner before we retired to the chalet. Despite being a married couple, Graham and I giggled like teenagers and were careful not to make any noise in our bedroom that might embarrass his parents – or ourselves.

'Are you happy?' Graham asked one night.

'Very,' I replied, gazing into his eyes. We'd both had too much sun and I probably should have been lying in a cool bath, but I clung to Graham's sunburnt body.

'About babies …' he said, looking lovingly into my eyes. 'When do you think …?'

'I'll qualify in December, all being well,' I mused. 'Then I will automatically get a staff post. After twelve months as a staff midwife I'll qualify as a sister …'

'A sister?' Graham asked anxiously, as if the idea had never occurred to him.

'Don't worry,' I soothed. 'I'm not trying to work my way up the ladder to become a Matron or anything like that. I'm not interested in delivering orders; I just want to deliver babies. It's simply the way the NHS works. It's a tiered system and it's just the next step along. I'd get more money and, eventually, a better shift pattern.'

Graham looked relieved. 'So how exactly does a family of our own fit into this plan?'

I wondered if his mum had been subtly asking the same thing, and I wouldn't have blamed her if she had. Graham was a year younger than me, but nevertheless I had to admit that at twenty-one and twenty-two we were approaching the time we would be expected to start thinking about having children.

'Let me see,' I teased. 'Staff midwife this year, sister by the end of 1971, then I'd need to find my feet in the job and … well, shall I pencil us in for, say, 1972 or 1973?'

'Done,' Graham said, kissing me.

Chapter Twelve

'Get these birds out of here, NOW!
Where's the hygiene? Tell me that?'

'I'm May Tattersall, pleased to meet you,'

It was July 1970 and I was going out for the very first time with community midwife Mrs Tattersall, my mentor for Part Two of my training.

'Pleased to meet you too,' I said, shaking her thin, outstretched hand.

Mrs Tattersall was a long-serving community midwife, and I knew she had an excellent reputation and was admired and respected by other members of staff. I'd seen her around the hospital many times and had been very much looking forward to meeting her. I was quite intrigued by her, actually, as from what I'd seen she didn't look as I'd imagined a middle-aged community midwife would. I think I expected someone matronly or perhaps more serene, with a sensible grey perm, but from a distance I had noted curiously that Mrs Tattersall was wire-thin and bottle blonde. What's more, she always appeared to be in a tearing hurry.

''Ow typical is that?' she said, peering through her black-rimmed spectacles at her notes. 'Your very first job in the community and it's out in t' middle o' bloody nowhere! Never mind, love, pick up that bag and come with me to the car. No doubt it'll be an education, this one.'

Her broad Manchester accent and the language she used took me by surprise, as did the state of her scuffed black lace-ups, which looked as if they'd never seen a brush or a tin of shoe polish, ever. Up close I could see that she had broken veins on her ruddy cheeks, and I could smell cigarettes on her breath.

Mrs Tattersall's dirty green Avenger, parked haphazardly across two spaces, was another eye-opener. I had to remove a pile of tatty magazines and a couple of chewed pencils from the front seat before I sat down, and I was astonished to see the ashtray was overflowing with cigarette ends. The smell of stale smoke clogged the air and a rotting apple core rolled around the foot-well in front of my seat. Mrs Tattersall didn't seem in the slightest bit bothered by this disarray and made no reference whatsoever to the state of the car.

'I've been up to this place several times, and it's always the bloody same,' she groaned. 'Flamin' animals running round all over t' place.'

We were headed for Ashton Moss, about three and a half miles away from the hospital on the outskirts of the town, heading towards Manchester. Maeve Blythe was expecting her fourth child and her husband Norris, a farmer, had walked two miles to the nearest phone box to telephone the hospital that morning. Mrs Tattersall explained this in between taking drags on a cigarette and grumbling 'Bloody hell!' at each red light and zebra crossing.

'Mr Blythe is noted for his fine turnips and cauliflowers, I'm led to believe, but they're a right daft pair,' she told me. 'Last time I visited, the mother-in-law was swinging a wedding ring over Mrs Blythe's belly saying, "'Appen it's another boy."'

'How could she tell?' I asked, naïvely.

'God only knows! I can't be doin' with those old wives' tales, they're a load of nonsense. Let that be your first lesson, Linda love. Don't bother askin' what it's all supposed to mean, and if they ask you, never get involved. It's your job to deal with what's real, not all that clap-trap. Whatever you tell them, they'll hang on your every word, so steer well clear, mark my words.'

'OK,' I said obediently. 'That sounds like a good idea.'

By the time we arrived at the run-down farmhouse I had really warmed to Mrs Tattersall. She might not fit the image of a senior midwife I'd been led to expect by my traditional training in Manchester, but she seemed laden with wisdom and I could tell there was a large, motherly heart inside her reedy body.

Mr Blythe greeted us at the gate. He was dressed in a mud-splattered shirt and dirty green wellingtons and was surrounded by three small boys in equally grubby, matching attire. There was a strong smell of manure in the air, and half a dozen scruffy hens were pecking noisily at the ground.

'She's in front room with Flora and Megan,' Mr Blythe said, pointing at the house. 'Please, go in, and I'll put t' kettle on.'

Mrs Tattersall gave me a look that said 'Oh dear, what did I tell you?' even though Mr Blythe had not yet, so far as I could tell, done anything to live up to his 'daft' reputation.

I helped Mrs Tattersall carry in the equipment, and we heard Mr Blythe call loudly to his wife: 'The midwife's here!' He sounded very relieved.

'Come in!' Mrs Blythe called out, sounding equally pleased at our arrival. We followed her voice into a large, hot and dusty room on the ground floor, where she lay on a high double bed that was covered with an assortment of hand-stitched quilts and crocheted blankets. Two Collie dogs lay either side of her, slathering and sniffing.

'You've met Flora and Megan before, haven't you?' she huffed politely to Mrs Tattersall, wincing slightly as a contraction rippled across her belly.

'Yes!' Mrs Tattersall replied rather sharply. 'But let's be having them off the bed while I examine you, shall we? This is Nurse Buckley, my assistant, by the way.'

I had imagined Flora and Megan to be a clucking mother and mother-in-law, or perhaps a couple of sisters, but certainly not a pair of lolloping farm dogs. I was astonished they were even in the room, let alone allowed up on the bed.

It turned out that Mrs Blythe's labour was already well established and, being her fourth child, it progressed very quickly. The dogs whimpered and whined each time they were batted away from the bed by Mrs Tattersall, and what with the noise of the now-squawking hens and the three excited lads playing tag in the yard outside the open window, we had a job hearing the nuances of Mrs Blythe's peculiarly controlled cries of 'oooumph' and 'yeeuuuurrr!'

Sometimes she gurned horribly when she cried out, which seemed to unsettle the dogs, and they both made repeated attempts to jump up and lick their mistress's face back to normal. I could see that Mrs Tattersall was getting increasingly irritated with the dogs' presence in the room, and when the pair of them started to sniff around the hem of Mrs Blythe's nightdress Mrs Tattersall nearly had a fit.

'Get down!' she spluttered. 'Be off with you!'

I was amazed she didn't just throw the animals out of the room and shut the door, but after her outburst she managed to bite her tongue as the labour continued to progress quite quickly. It was only when Mr Blythe appeared with another cup of tea for us all, just minutes before his fourth son burst triumphantly into the world, that Mrs Tattersall finally exploded once and for all.

Two scraggy hens had followed Mr Blythe into the room, and they strutted straight over to Mrs Tattersall squawking loudly, with chests puffed out as if they owned the place.

'Enough!' Mrs Tattersall bellowed. 'Mr Blythe, please get these birds out of here, NOW! Where's the hygiene? Tell me that? Where's the hygiene? OUT! NOW!'

The poor man was taken aback at his telling off and began to chase the hens around the room in his haste to obey, leaving clumps of manure-scented mud across the carpet as he did so. Baby Blythe, a magnificent boy weighing almost ten pounds, was delivered in the midst of this chaos onto a quilt covered in dog hairs, to the sound of shouting and screeching that had nothing to do with his mother.

'Could you not have insisted on taking the dogs out of the room?' I asked Mrs Tattersall later.

'Well,' she said, in a voice laden with prudence, 'it's like this. When you're a community midwife, you have to fit in with the community. Women who want to have their baby at home usually do so because they feel more comfortable in their home environment than in the clinical surroundings of a maternity hospital. It's our job to fit in with them, not the other way around. If she wants her dogs there, then it's best to try to accommodate her, as far as possible.'

'But … not hens?'

'Not hens, no, never hens,' Mrs Tattersall said firmly.

I expected some pearls of wisdom about the dangers of toxoplasmosis or even salmonella poisoning, but Mrs Tattersall simply said with a rasp: 'I flamin' well hate birds!'

On the way back we called in to see Mrs Shawcross, who lived in a tiny terraced house close to the hospital. She had given birth to a little boy called Stanley the previous week, and Mrs Tattersall wanted to check that all was well. In those days, new mothers were visited by a community midwife every day for the first ten days after a home birth.

'She's a nice young girl, seems a bit anxious though,' Mrs Tattersall told me. 'It's her first baby.'

Mrs Shawcross answered the door in her dressing gown, though it was now the afternoon. She had black circles under her eyes and looked utterly exhausted. We had to squeeze past a pram and bike that cluttered the hallway before finding baby Stanley sleeping soundly in a Moses basket on the floor of the cramped living room. Mrs Shawcross had clearly been dozing on the settee close to her son, but she nevertheless welcomed us warmly and began plumping up the cushions and removing a newspaper and a pile of cloth nappies from the seats, urging us to sit down in comfort.

When Mrs Shawcross went to put the kettle on, Mrs Tattersall had a quick look at Stanley, then said to me, 'Get used to this, Linda. People treat midwives like local dignitaries! Quite flattering, I suppose.'

Mrs Shawcross reappeared with a tray of tea served in what must have been her best china cups and saucers. There was also a small glass on the tray, containing a purple-coloured liquid. 'Stanley seems to like a bit of Vimto on his dummy,' Mrs Shawcross said by way of explanation, gesturing towards the glass.

Mrs Tattersall shot a glance at Stanley, who had a large blue plastic dummy in his mouth. 'Perhaps that isn't a good idea,' Mrs Tatterhall said tactfully. 'Vimto's not made for babies, you see. May I ask, did you put it on neat?'

'Oh yes, I did. He didn't like it diluted. He only settles when we give it to him neat.'

'Well, I don't think you've done him any harm, but let's not give Stanley any more Vimto, shall we not?'

'Right you are,' Mrs Shawcross immediately agreed. 'I probably wasn't thinking straight, I'm so short of sleep.'

I loved the way Mrs Tattersall handled the situation. There was no embarrassment or chastisement; she had delivered her professional advice tactfully yet authoritatively, and Mrs Shawcross wasn't in the slightest bit put out.

'I can see for myself that you're looking ever so tired,' Mrs Tattersall went on. 'How is Stanley sleeping at night?'

'Not brilliant, as he doesn't like sleeping upstairs,' Mrs Shawcross said flatly. 'Last night he just wouldn't settle at all. We were up and down to him for hours, so we brought him downstairs. My husband eventually managed to get him to sleep on a blanket on the rug here, so we brought our bedding downstairs and slept beside him.'

I could hear Mrs Tattersall drawing in a long breath before telling Mrs Shawcross that perhaps this wasn't such a good idea either.

'It's like this,' she said patiently. 'Stanley probably doesn't know whether he's upstairs, downstairs or in m'Lady's chamber for that matter, but he will certainly sense that his parents are getting a bit anxious about him. Take my advice and don't sleep on the floor with Stanley again. Stay in your own bed where you will feel more comfortable, and try not to fret.

Stanley will settle better when you and your husband are more relaxed. How does that sound?'

'Right you are,' Mrs Shawcross said again. 'Do you know, sometimes you can't see the wood for the trees when you're short of sleep, can you?'

On the pavement outside, Mrs Tattersall raised her eyebrows to the sky. 'God help them, whatever next!'

'Couldn't she give the baby gripe water to help him settle?' I enquired.

'She could eventually, if colic is the problem, though it's too early to tell and you don't give it until the baby is at least a month old,' Mrs Tattersall replied. 'But in my experience gripe water works very well. I think it's probably the alcohol in it that does the trick. Vimto indeed! Whatever was she thinking, giving a baby something so sugary!'

That night Graham lapped up my stories. He laughed his head off when I told him about the chickens at baby Blythe's birth and he couldn't believe that the entire Shawcross family had slept on the floor together because of seven-day-old Stanley.

'I love being out in the community,' I told him. 'It's such an eye-opener.'

'You can say that again,' Graham chuckled. 'And I can see a change in you.'

'How do you mean?'

'You're enjoying yourself,' he replied. 'You don't seem nervous or daunted at all, yet you're doing what's effectively a brand new job. It's as if you were made for this. I'm ever so pleased for you.'

Graham's words rang true. I felt I could really be myself with Mrs Tattersall, and over the coming weeks and months I looked forward to every day spent with her. She was a real, down-to-earth human being, and a very caring one at that. Funnily enough, I can't say I got to know a great deal about her personal life. I knew she had two sons and some grandchildren and lived over by the Army barracks about half a mile from the hospital, but she wasn't a great talker. Whenever we were together her focus was on the task in hand. I guessed she was in her late forties or early fifties, but I wasn't sure and would certainly never have asked her anything like that. Likewise, I could never have called her May in a million years; she was always Mrs Tattersall to me.

In time I began to get to know how Mrs Tattersall's mind worked, and I was constantly impressed by how very skilled she was at her job. I saw the way she expertly scanned the room whenever we walked into someone's home, taking in much more than the mother and baby she had come to visit.

'I've got some liquid here to put on their hair,' she often said, after watching a young child scratch its head, then she would gently enquire about nits at the local school. Everything she said sounded matter-of-fact, and nobody ever took offence.

'Have you finished with that other carrycot?' she would ask if she spotted a new one in a house. 'Only I know a family who could get some use out of that ...'

We often left our routine visits carting out old baby baths or high chairs that might 'do' for somebody else, and people were always willing to help and share. Everybody seemed to respect and admire Mrs Tattersall for showing such generous community spirit.

On one occasion I was shocked to hear my mentor ask a new young father, 'Have you got enough to eat?' Ashton and its surrounding area were neither deprived nor wealthy. Men tended to do blue-collar jobs, typically working as tradesmen, bus drivers or for companies like the local electricity board, Norweb. I had never heard of anyone going hungry, but Mrs Tattersall knew the young man had lost his job recently and money was tight.

'We're getting by,' came the dignified reply.

The next time we passed the house Mrs Tattersall had loaded the car with goodies, which she delivered to this man's grateful wife, completely without ceremony.

'Here, one of my colleagues was baking last night and she gave me these buns and a milk pudding. I won't use them – will you?'

The woman beamed appreciatively as we drove quickly away. It was classic Mrs Tattersall.

Nothing seemed to faze her, and I felt able to ask her most questions that popped into my head, without feeling embarrassed.

'What's "payment in kind"?' I asked one day. I had heard two midwives discussing a patient who had given birth at the hospital a few days earlier. I gathered that the married young woman had decided to have her baby adopted because of this 'payment in kind' problem, and I didn't understand it.

'Linda, love, I know the girl you're talking about. It's like this. She slept with her landlord because she and her husband couldn't afford to pay the rent. It was either that or be thrown out on the streets. Sadly, the young woman fell pregnant, with the landlord being the father of the baby.'

I was horrified. I'd been shocked by the stories of the prostitutes I'd heard at St Mary's but I was absolutely stunned that such a sordid arrangement could take place right here on my own doorstep.

'So that's why she is having the baby adopted,' I gasped, the penny slowly dropping. I knew that babies who were being put up for adoption were removed from their mothers as swiftly as possible after the birth. The poor women weren't allowed to hold their babies, even for a minute. This was the kindest way, it was thought, as it stopped the mother becoming attached to her child, and would help her cope with the separation.

'What will happen to that girl now?' I asked.

'Her husband is letting her stay, I believe. He said she could stay but the baby had to go, so I hear.'

That was the end of the conversation. Mrs Tattersall always gave straight answers, but she wasn't one to gossip. I liked that. I was learning so much from her, things you couldn't possibly have learned from a midwifery textbook.

Despite being exposed to some of life's tough realities, I was in my element. I aspired to be as good and experienced a midwife as Mrs Tattersall, and I watched and listened eagerly each and every day, lapping up everything she said and did, and feeling privileged to be her pupil.

Chapter Thirteen

'So you've had the baby? ... Let's have a
cup of tea and a cigarette then'

One night in September 1970, when I was in the third month
of Part Two of my training, Mrs Tattersall and I were brewing
a pot of tea in the nurses' kitchen when we were called out to
a delivery.

'Bloody hell, why do these women always leave it till an
ungodly hour to go into labour?' Mrs Tattersall rasped. 'And
will you look at the night!'

I looked out of the rain-splattered window as Mrs Tattersall
stubbed out her cigarette in the sink. It sizzled when it made
contact with dregs of cold tea, no doubt discarded by the last
midwives to have their break interrupted.

It certainly was a filthy night outside. Mrs Tattersall and I
had not long returned from checking up on another expectant
mother, and the weather had closed in. The sky was as black
as the ace of spades and thick curtains of drizzle were clearly
visible beneath the streetlights.

'Want a lift or will you take the scooter?'

'I'll take the scooter. I'll see you there,' I smiled, thinking of
the lipstick-stained fag ends that littered the floor of Mrs
Tattersall's Avenger and deciding that despite the rain I'd
rather ride my moped. With its small 50cc engine it was officially a moped, not a scooter, though I would never have
corrected Mrs Tattersall.

I pulled on my blue NHS-issue raincoat to protect my uniform from the rain, took out my bun, which was held in place by a little blue velvet ribbon over a rubber band, and headed out into the night.

As I pulled on my crash helmet I ran through a mental checklist. Mrs Tattersall had visited Mrs Willis last week, two weeks before the baby's due date, to deposit vital equipment. There would be two sets of Spencer Wells forceps, the same as ones we used in the hospital, a pair of scissors and a roll of cotton wool already waiting for us.

Tonight, Mrs Tattersall would bring a kidney-shaped receiver dish in which to collect the placenta, scales to weigh the baby, a Pinard stethoscope to monitor the heartbeat and a sphygmomanometer to test the mother's blood pressure. All I needed were my notes and, most importantly, a Jacob's Tea Cake to stop me fainting with hunger. I'd learned by now that expectant dads are absolutely brilliant at making cups of tea, but they never, ever offered us midwives anything to eat.

I checked my coat pocket for both the notebook and the biscuit and set off into the darkness with Mrs Tattersall's directions ringing in my head.

'Straight over at the junction, keep left until you pass the bus shelter and keep your eyes peeled for Willshaw Lane, for goodness sake. It's easily missed in this bloody rain!'

I must remember to put the Tea Cake discreetly in my uniform pocket before I enter the house, I thought, then I could eat it when I nip to the bathroom later.

'Must think we run on thin air!' Mrs Tattersall frequently complained, though I never saw her eat a thing as she seemed to prefer a cigarette to a snack.

As my trusty moped slowly but surely carried me to Willshaw Lane I ran another mental checklist through my head, this time taking stock of my own life.

I was in the final stage of my midwifery training. I had three hard years of nurses' training behind me and had passed Part One of my ten-month-long midwifery course with flying colours. Now, at the tender age of twenty-two, I was out in the community, well on my way to completing Part Two, which would make me a qualified midwife at last. I could feel my confidence growing daily, and I felt lucky to be learning from a professional like Mrs Tattersall.

I felt a rush of excitement, even though the rain was now spiking my cheeks like cold needles. This part of the job was exhilarating. I felt important, riding through the night to the aid of a pregnant woman. I wasn't afraid, as I didn't yet have the responsibility of delivering a baby all by myself, but I was *that* close, and was finally starting to feel like a proper little midwife.

I was glad to see that Mrs Tattersall had beaten me to the semi-detached house, but nevertheless when the expectant father answered my knock at the door he gave me a broad, relieved smile. It was a look I was beginning to know well, and I liked it.

'The midwife's here!' he almost sang as he welcomed me in. When his wife is in labour, it was becoming apparent, there are no more comforting words a man can utter.

Mrs Willis was labouring on a bed that had been brought down to the lounge so as not to disturb her two young sons who were sleeping upstairs. It was 11.30 p.m. and she'd been in slow labour for a few hours already, but was clearly coping very well.

'Thanks for coming,' she smiled as she fished in her hand-bag for a Spangle sweet to suck on. 'I feel better now you're both here.'

From past experience I knew Mrs Tattersall would not have made a song and dance about the fact I was still a student, as that might alarm the patient. I would simply have been introduced as 'Nurse Linda Buckley', possibly with the words 'my colleague' tagged on the end, which gave me a flush of pride.

I surveyed the room. A brown-and-cream striped settee and armchair had been pushed back against the far wall to make way for the bed, which was covered in a very fashionable spiral-patterned quilt. I'd seen a similar one on display in the window of Marshall & Snelgrove in the centre of Manchester recently, so I knew it was all the rage and had probably cost a pretty penny. I was concerned the quilt would get ruined.

'Don't worry, Derek has seen to it that we have plenty of towels,' Mrs Willis said, noticing me looking at her bed linen. 'And there's a towel and a piece of soap laid out for you in the bathroom, Nurse.'

I felt very important, being welcomed into the Willis's home on such a momentous day in their lives. Two bars of an electric fire glowed orange in the hearth, which was surrounded by an elaborate brick fireplace covering an entire wall of the sitting room. On the mantelpiece were displayed several souvenir plates from holidays in Prestatyn and Rhyl, depicting painted scenes of caravan parks and donkeys on the beach.

'Linda, please see to it that the instruments are sterilised,' Mrs Tattersall instructed. 'Mr Willis will provide you with a pan.'

I followed Mr Willis into the kitchen, where a large stainless-steel pressure-cooker pan was standing on the Formica worktop.

'I hope it's big enough; it's the biggest we have,' he apologised.

'It's perfect,' I assured him, and indeed it was.

I remembered Mrs Tattersall's words of wisdom as I shifted the pan onto the hob and struck a match to light the gas.

'Sterility is not the be all and end all,' she had told me. 'Remember, the instruments have already been cleaned at the hospital. It is our job to make sure they are "socially clean". By that I mean they are as clean as we can possibly get them in the circumstances. At the end of the day, any germs that are knocking about are the mother's own germs, because we are in her house. Just do your best.'

Mrs Tattersall examined Mrs Willis while I boiled up the forceps and scissors. Mr Willis busied himself in the kitchen, too, as it wasn't the done thing for men to get in the way during an examination.

'We could have hours yet, but you're doing well,' I heard Mrs Tattersall wheeze.

Mr Willis made us all a cup of tea and we settled around the bed, chatting softly and pausing to offer words of comfort and encouragement whenever a contraction made Mrs Willis wince.

Mrs Tattersall made a note of the time, followed by the scribbled observation 'five centimetres dilated', which she let me see but did not discuss with Mrs Willis. In those days women rarely asked questions and didn't expect to be given medical details; they simply put their faith in their midwife and did as they were told. It was almost unprecedented for a woman to have read a book about pregnancy, and I had even heard midwives telling patients not to bother looking at what scant leaflets there were at the antenatal clinic, remarking that it might not do them any good to 'know too much'.

Mrs Tattersall put down her brief notes and began circling letters in a word search puzzle in her *People's Friend* magazine.

'I'd play a record but I'm afraid of waking the little 'uns upstairs,' Mr Willis said earnestly.

'My wife likes The Beatles. Do you?'

'Oh yes, I do,' I smiled. 'John Lennon is my idol, he's *my* Beatle. I saw them live at the Apollo in Ardwick in 1965.'

'Never! You lucky duck!' exclaimed Mrs Willis, with such vigour she brought on her biggest contraction yet.

'Tell me all about it,' she panted, clutching her stomach and wrinkling her brow until the pain subsided.

'Well, I nagged my dad to give me a lift up to the Apollo at 5.30 a.m. on the day the tickets went on sale,' I said. 'I remember I took a hard-boiled egg in my pocket in case I got hungry, but I was too excited to think about eating it. I felt like I'd won the Pools when I got my hands on that little yellow ticket. It cost me 15 shillings, and was the best thing I had ever bought in my life! My school friend Susan Thornley was with me, and we hugged each other and jumped up and down, we were so thrilled.'

Mrs Willis took a sharp intake of breath. 'Hold my hand, Derek, this is a big one coming,' she gasped.

'Go on, Nurse, keep talking, please tell me moooore,' she implored, the word morphing into the sound of a mooing cow.

I glanced at Mrs Tattersall, who gave me an encouraging nod.

'I can't remember much about the music,' I went on. 'I don't think I heard a thing. I just screamed and screamed, because that's what everyone else did ...'

Bang on cue Mrs Willis let out an ear-piercing shriek.

'Oooh heck, that was a big one,' she puffed. 'Sorry about that.'

'We don't mind the noise, but make sure you don't hurt your throat,' I smiled. 'I don't want you ending up like me after that concert. My throat was so swollen from all the screaming I couldn't talk for days afterwards!'

And so the night went on, and on.

We chatted in a friendly but polite way, drank lots of tea and watched and listened as Mrs Willis, who eventually asked me to call her Brenda, huffed and occasionally screamed through her slow and steady labour.

At 7.30 a.m. Mrs Tattersall wrote up some notes, stood up suddenly and announced, 'I'm going out to find a telephone.'

I followed her to the door anxiously as she pulled on her coat.

'We're never going to make the 8.30 a.m. clinic at this rate,' she complained, rolling her eyes to the ceiling.

Seeing my own eyes widen to the size of dinner plates, she added, 'You'll be absolutely fine, Linda. I won't be long. I expect she's got a way to go yet.'

Mr and Mrs Willis didn't seem the slightest bit perturbed by Mrs Tattersall's departure, but I was too busy fretting about being left alone and in charge to feel flattered by their reaction.

'There's a phone box down Wood Lane I used to call you from last night,' Mr Willis instructed helpfully as he saw her out. 'I'll put another brew on when you get back.'

I pulled up a brown leather pouffe to the side of the bed and patted Mrs Willis's hand. 'It's been a long night. How are you feeling?' I asked.

'I think I want to push,' came the unexpected reply.

My pulse quickened but I didn't flinch as I hastily adjusted her nightgown and bedclothes and prepared to examine her.

'Oh, right you are. Deep breaths. Remember what we've taught you. Take your time …'

'The baby's coming!' she panted. 'It's coming right now!'

'I'm right here. You're doing fine, Mrs Willis,' I said, ignoring the static shock that crackled up the back of my stocking as I knelt on the thick nylon rug at the end of the bed. Mr Willis hurried out of the room in the direction of the kitchen.

'I can see the baby's head,' I said, surprised at how calm my voice sounded. 'You're doing magnificently, Brenda. One more push should do it … go on now!'

I saw the baby give a little turn as it plopped out perfectly onto the chocolate-brown towels Mr Willis had laid beneath his wife.

'Well done!' I exclaimed, as much to myself as to Mrs Willis. 'It's a girl, a beautiful little girl!' I picked her up and she let out a mighty cry.

Mr Willis crept gingerly into the room and kissed his wife on her flushed red cheeks, while I cut the umbilical cord and watched the proud parents breathe a delighted sigh of relief.

The baby looked completely adorable and I was thrilled at the sight of her too, but I couldn't allow myself to relax and celebrate until the placenta was delivered. Only then could I be sure that Mrs Willis wouldn't haemorrhage, and my job would be done.

Without delay, I injected Mrs Willis with Syntometrine. I'd already prepared it, thinking at the time that it might be my only hands-on role in the birth, with Mrs Tattersall in charge. As I gave the injection in her thigh I explained to Mrs Willis with as much authority as I could muster that it was to help her expel the placenta. I made myself smile brightly at her, wanting to reassure her that I was completely in control of the situation, even though I was thinking to myself, 'Stay calm. This is still not over. I'm not in the hospital now; I'm in an ordinary house. I have no oxygen on the wall, no buzzer to press if things go wrong.'

Thankfully, Mrs Willis delivered the placenta with impressive ease and was so preoccupied with gazing at her new daughter I don't think she'd have picked up on my underlying anxiety even if I'd been dripping with sweat and shaking from head to foot with nerves. I proceeded to clean the little girl and weigh her before putting on a terry towelling nappy and white cotton nightdress and laying her in the waiting crib beside her mother. I did this swiftly and efficiently, wanting to finish the job professionally, and I felt a fabulous warm glow spreading around my body. 'I did it!' I thought to myself, an involuntary, genuine grin spreading across my face. *'I've* done this!'

I will never forget the overwhelming feelings of relief and sheer, unbridled delight I experienced in that front room. The baby's warm skin and soft downy head, the tiny bubbles of saliva that popped daintily on her lips as she let out her first cry, and the minute, shell-like fingernails on the tips of her wriggling fingers all captivated me. I'd brought a new life into the world! I was sure I couldn't have felt happier if I were Mrs Willis herself, and she was indeed a picture of pure joy and triumph.

All that remained was for me to record the delivery time and birth details in my notes. While I did so, Mr Willis fetched his two young sons from upstairs and they scampered with great excitement into the sitting room to meet their little sister.

'Meet Lorinda Louise,' Mr Willis beamed.

Stepping back, I felt incredibly satisfied as I took my pen from my apron pocket and proudly recorded the time of the textbook delivery as 7.45 a.m. precisely.

I looked at the Willis family. They were all quiet now, gazing at Lorinda Louise in awe.

'Aren't we lucky to have a little girl?' Mrs Willis beamed as she admired her sleeping daughter, who was snugly wrapped in a hand-crocheted yellow blanket. 'If we'd known I'd have got Nana to knit that in pink!'

She turned to me and said, 'Thank you, Nurse. You were marvellous! I couldn't have done it without you. Thank you so much!'

The big brothers, dressed in matching Thunderbirds pyjamas, began to jostle for prime position at the side of the crib, elbowing each other but never once taking their eyes off their new little sister. The entire family could not have looked happier if they tried.

The magnitude of the occasion hit me with even greater force. I hadn't just delivered a baby; I'd performed a miracle! Lorinda Louise was the very first baby I had delivered all by myself! There was no qualified midwife guiding my hands, as I was used to. I was out in the community on my own, and I'd done it without so much as a whisper from my mentor. I didn't have Sister Houghton's hands to guide me and I didn't have Mrs Tattersall by my side. All my training and hard work had paid dividends. This was the very best feeling in the world, ever. Midwifery was my vocation, and I could actually do it! I *had* done it! I'd delivered a baby – me, Linda Buckley!

A knock at the door interrupted my triumphant thoughts.

'Eee, it's brass monkeys out there,' I heard Mrs Tattersall exclaim loudly as Mr Willis let her in. I noticed it was 8.30 a.m., and it was only then that it dawned on me she had been gone a full hour.

Mr Willis was grinning like a Cheshire cat, and Mrs Tattersall knew the look of a proud new father when she saw one.

'So you've had the baby?' Mrs Tattersall said in a kindly tone as she crossed the sitting room and peered in the cot. 'Oh, that's good. Let's have a cup of tea and a cigarette then.'

Mr Willis obliged yet again with the tea and Mr and Mrs Willis and Mrs Tattersall each lit up a cigarette from a packet of John Player's No. 6. All three proceeded to smoke contentedly around the sleeping baby.

I sipped my tea quietly, taking in the scene before me. I was surrounded by clouds of smoke and I was floating on cloud nine. I felt like shouting out: 'How can you all act so normal? I've just performed an absolute miracle and look at you puffing on your cigarettes!'

I didn't, of course. I dutifully helped pack the equipment away, said my goodbyes and rode my moped back to the hospital, where I was expected to carry on with clinic duties. Normally I'd have been dead on my legs after working all through the night, but I was buzzing with the thrill of my first solo delivery.

'So you've got your "confidence case" nicely under your belt,' Mrs Tattersall smiled later, when I was called to her office to receive my report.

I'd heard the term many times before, but only now did I fully appreciate its meaning. I was brimming with confidence, that's for sure, and I couldn't wait for my next delivery.

'I think you'll find I've given you a very good report,' Mrs Tattersall said, passing me a brown folder. This was a record that had to be written up by the mentor whenever a pupil midwife delivered a baby. 'You thoroughly deserve it, Linda. Well done, love.'

I never did find out what took her so long when she went to the telephone box, and I never asked.

'Maybe the clever fox knew quite well what would happen,' I said to Graham later that day. 'I wouldn't put it past her.'

'She wouldn't have taken any chances if she didn't have complete faith in you,' he replied, pulling me in for a cuddle. 'I've always said you're a natural. I'm so proud of you, my little nurse.'

Graham always drew out the letters of the word 'n-u-r-s-e' when he called me that, as if softly savouring the sound.

'I'm a midwife now ... well, very nearly. You'll soon have to call me "my little m-i-d-w-i-f-e" instead.'

It thrilled me to think I would soon become a fully qualified midwife, and I kissed Graham and thanked him for all his support over the years.

'I wouldn't have got this far without you,' I told him.

'Course you would!' he smiled. 'It's your calling!'

'I mean it,' I replied. 'It's been really tough, tougher than I ever imagined. Without your support I would have quit years ago.'

Later that same week Mrs Tattersall rushed purposefully along the hospital corridor towards me. It was Saturday night, she had a delivery bag in one hand and a packet of cigarettes in the other, and I could see we had another birth to dash to. I immediately felt excited, but my heart sank like a stone when she said, 'Meet me at Moira Petty's on Hope Street.'

I'd been to the Petty house several times before, and of all the homes I'd visited this was the only one that pushed me right out of my comfort zone. Moira lived with her mum and two sisters. Each of the girls, all in their late teens or early twenties at most, had two children. This would be Moira's third baby, making it the seventh infant in a house that was already bursting at the seams.

The house was filthy and damp. The first time I did a home visit I was horrified to see several dirty mattresses leaning up against the walls in the back dining room. Mrs Tattersall explained that there were so many people living under the one roof, and one of the rooms was so damp upstairs, that the sisters and their children had to sleep downstairs. This meant when they needed the space during the day they just propped up their mattresses.

The air was permanently thick with the pungent smell of sweaty, dirty bodies. Children with scraggy hair and grimy faces scampered about in vests and sagging nappies, and a scruffy black dog stuck its nose into everything and appeared to be the family's only means of cleaning the tiled floor in the back room, where the girls slept. I say this because on my first visit a few weeks earlier, one of the sisters knocked a box containing two eggs off the dining table, which stood in the centre of the room. Both eggs smashed on the quarry tiles, making a huge mess, but nobody attempted to clean it up. I soon realised why not, when the hungry hound ran in and gobbled up not only the broken eggs but their shells too, licking the floor so clean the only evidence he left was the empty egg box.

Even on a bright day it was always dark and cold in the house, and the family had no hot water. 'We won't have a cup of tea,' Mrs Tattersall had said as we pulled up outside on that very first visit, and I understood why as soon as we stepped inside. I had never encountered a family as poverty-stricken as the Pettys, and their lifestyle shocked and upset me. It wasn't just the dirt and the fact they were obviously very poor that was so distressing; it was that none of the girls seemed to have any purpose to their life. They were just surviving, producing babies they had no means of supporting. Their world was as far away from my own as I could imagine.

'How can they live like that?' I asked Mrs Tattersall one day. 'I know they have no money, but I don't understand why they don't even wash themselves. I mean, they must know they smell awful.'

'Some people don't know any different,' she explained plainly. 'If your mum's never taught you how to wash properly, you don't learn, do you? They will never have seen their mum brush her teeth or keep herself clean, so they don't know any other way of being. They have no hot water, so God only knows it would be hard enough for them even if they knew what they were doing.'

The Petty family's circumstances were by no means typical of the area. There was industrial unrest grumbling away in some parts of Britain, but here in Ashton, from what I saw, life generally seemed to trundle on regardless and most people got by and certainly didn't live below the breadline. I had seen some worrying reports on the news about job losses and fears of wage cuts amongst postal workers and miners elsewhere in the country. Closer to home, the local Granada Television workers were planning strike action, complaining about pay and refusing to work with colour television equipment. I remember that clearly as there was talk that some episodes of *Coronation Street* might have to be recorded in black and white again, instead of the new colour that everyone was raving about.

However, as far as I knew, none of these issues affected the Petty household. The Pettys were not victims of the economy or social change. Instead, it seemed they chose to live the way they did, scraping by with what little money they were given in state hand-outs because they didn't appear to know any better.

The home visits prior to the birth were a huge eye-opener for me and I didn't enjoy them one bit, but Mrs Tattersall always made sure I accompanied her. I didn't fully realise until the night of the actual delivery that she had done it to prepare me and cushion me from the shock in advance.

When we met outside the house at 10 p.m. I was shivering.

'Ready?' Mrs Tattersall asked with a reassuring look after I had parked my moped and pulled off my helmet.

'I am,' I nodded. Thanks to Mrs Tattersall I was shivering more from the cold wind that was blowing than through nerves this time.

'That's good,' she said. 'I need you to be focused on mother and baby tonight, nothing else.'

Hauling her bag of instruments out of the boot of her car, Mrs Tattersall continued in a voice loud enough to be heard down the street, 'I hope the lover's not here. That bloody man gets right up my nose. We could do without him swaggering around drunk, getting in the way.'

I'd never met the man myself and had no idea what his name was, and I don't think Mrs Tattersall did either as she only ever referred to him as 'the lover'. All I knew was that he was Moira's mum's boyfriend, and according to Mrs Tattersall he appeared to be the only man to have anything to do with the household. She had it on good authority he was in trouble with the police and only ever went out at night, under cover of darkness, when he snuck to the local pub and staggered home blind drunk at closing time. His police record meant he couldn't work, or so the story went, and we could only presume he lived on the state benefits claimed by the women. Mrs Tattersall clearly didn't see fit to delve any deeper into the family set-up, and I trusted her instincts.

I dearly hoped he wasn't home and was relieved when one of Moira's sisters answered the door and showed us into the front room, which the family referred to as the parlour. This was the best room in the house, and as such was usually reserved for the mother and her lover. Moira must have been given special permission to use it tonight. She was lying down on a saggy mattress in the middle of the floor, surrounded by an assortment of grubby, threadbare towels and blankets.

My heart went out to her. She was wearing an old skirt and had bare legs that looked grey with cold and dirt. Mrs Tattersall examined her and remarked it was lucky she'd brought the instruments already sterilised, as labour was very well established and the baby could arrive before midnight.

'Let's hope so,' she whispered to me under her breath. 'The lover's at the pub. It would be good to get this baby out before he rolls in.'

I thought so too. I wasn't used to seeing people drunk and I felt anxious in this house late at night and wanted to go home as quickly as possible.

It was an uneventful, routine labour. Moira was courageous in the face of her contractions, making relatively little noise and following Mrs Tattersall's instructions carefully with regards to breathing correctly and shifting her position on the mattress when it would make her more comfortable.

'It will be time to push very soon, I think,' Mrs Tattersall advised. 'But don't push until I tell you, Moira. You know that, don't you?'

Moira nodded. 'I've done it twice before,' she said, 'and it weren't that long ago. I've not forgotten, Nurse.'

The dog barking manically in the hallway alerted us to the sound of the front door opening.

'Will ya mind me bleeding coat,' Mrs Petty slurred. 'You'll be yanking it right off me arm, ya big oaf!'

Moments later the parlour door swung open and the lover stood swaying dangerously before us. He was a dead ringer for Stan Ogden in *Coronation Street*, and Mrs Petty didn't look too dissimilar to Hilda Ogden with her headscarf and red lipstick, which was painted on in a thin bow shape that didn't match the size of her lips.

The pair of them stank of alcohol and appeared too drunk to register what was happening to Moira. I felt sick to my stomach and my legs started to twitch and jump involuntarily with nerves. It had never happened to me before, but I simply couldn't stop my legs from jangling.

'What's she doin' in here?' the lover bawled, waving his finger towards poor Moira.

'Baby's on it's way, ya daft fool,' Moira's mum chided, as the penny dropped.

'Well, I'm having the parlour!' he grunted.

Mrs Tattersall sprang towards him immediately and stood taller than I had ever seen her, hands on hips and chin jutted forward.

'I'm afraid you can't come in,' she said firmly.

'Who the 'ell are you to tell me what to do?'

'The midwife, for your information. Moira here is in labour. Now if you don't mind, sir …'

The lover took a step forward and pushed his jowly face towards Mrs Tattersall's.

'But I want to come in here,' he implored, sounding more pathetic than menacing now. 'I just want to come in t'parlour and sit down …'

He was rocking from side to side as he spoke and his speech was so slack it was as if he'd been punched in the face and his jaw was unhinged.

Moira's mum just gaped and stood rooted to the spot, making no attempt to stop her boyfriend as he lunged haphazardly forward once more.

Mrs Tattersall snapped in frustration. 'Get out of this parlour NOW!' she yelled, sounding more like a fishwife than a professional midwife. 'Go on, move it! Get out of here!'

With that she literally pushed the lover out the door. Moira's mum staggered out behind him and Mrs Tattersall closed the door firmly. 'Good riddance,' I wanted to say, and I knew that was exactly what Mrs Tattersall was thinking. Rubbing her hands together and smoothing down her apron, she went briskly back to attend to Moira, who was smiling sweetly and thanking her.

'There now, where were we before we were rudely interrupted?' Mrs Tattersall asked calmly, and order was magically restored.

I still felt on edge, but thanks to Mrs Tattersall my nerves were no longer fraught, and I felt a little less sick inside.

I delivered Moira's baby, a little boy she named Jimmy, just before 1 a.m. It was a straightforward birth and, despite our grim surroundings, when I held the baby I felt the same incredible surge of exhilaration I'd experienced when I brought Lorinda Louise into the world. After I'd cleaned Jimmy up as best I could with some water boiled in a battered old metal pan, I was delighted to see Moira had a new set of clothes for him.

I dressed him in the little white vest, white knitted trousers and a pale yellow matinée jacket, which Moira told me had been made by a kindly old neighbour. Moira's two sisters and her mother, who had sobered up considerably by now, all came to have a look at the new addition to the family.

'Look at you, gorgeous – another flamin' mouth to feed!' one sister said as she gazed lovingly at her new nephew.

'What are we going to do with you then, little Jimmy?' asked the other sister. 'We're outnumbered now, girls, that's for sure!'

There were no complications, and Mrs Tattersall and I left around 3 a.m.

'I'm so glad he had a new set of clothes,' I remarked as we stepped on to the pitch-black street outside. It was the only positive thing I could think of to say about the family.

'Linda, love, they will be the only new clothes that child will ever have,' Mrs Tattersall sniffed. 'And I can guarantee that before we've turned the corner of Hope Street, Moira will be out of that parlour as quick as you like so the lover can install his fat backside in the best chair as per usual.'

I don't know if that's actually what happened on the night she gave birth, but when I returned for a home visit a few days later Moira was indeed crammed in the back room again with her sisters and their seven young children. I had never seen any evidence of them cooking a meal during any of my visits, and the children seemed to survive on unbuttered buns, which their mothers dished out and let them roam around with, scattering crumbs on the floor that the dog wolfed down. My heart ached for Moira, but I tried to take comfort from the fact little Jimmy was in fine fettle in spite of his desperate surroundings.

'I'm afraid it's not your job to get involved in the whys and wherefores,' Mrs Tattersall told me when Moira was discharged from our care a few weeks later. 'That family is very unusual in these parts, thank God. It's a crying shame for those girls, but our job is done. We've delivered her baby safely, Moira has no ongoing complications and we've dished out all the advice we can.'

I knew this was true, and I took some solace from Mrs Tattersall's experienced words. Moira had been told how to boil up the bottles and teats in a pan before filling them with warm milk. The milk should be squirted onto the inside of the wrist to test it was not too hot or too cold, I told her. I also gave instructions about soaking cloth nappies overnight in a bucket before washing them out, and keeping the baby's bottom clean so as to avoid nappy rash.

Moira nodded obediently but I knew full well the family did not even own a bath, and the other children in the house wore dirty nappies, scratched their heads because of the lice and smelled absolutely awful.

When I returned to my own home that night, I found a note on the kitchen worktop from Graham, who had gone out to the pub for the evening with some friends. It read: 'Your mum brought a steak pie for tomorrow and some parkin. Are you off next Friday and if so shall we go to The Sportsman for a meal? Love you, sleep tight.' I felt almost guilty, having so much when the Pettys had so little, and I understood exactly why Mrs Tattersall often helped poor families with gifts of food and baby equipment.

This feeling stayed with me and was intensified two days later when my father came round to deliver the most wonderful news. My brother John and his wife Nevim had become the proud parents of a healthy little boy they named Kerem. He was born on Monday 7 September 1970 by Caesarean section at a hospital in Brussels, where my brother and sister-in-law were now happily living and working.

'Shame you weren't on hand, Linda,' Dad smiled. 'I expect they could have used your skills!'

I'd heard variations on this comment for months now, ever since we discovered Nevim was pregnant. Everybody I told about the baby asked me, 'Oooh, will you be their midwife?' to which I always laughed and explained that they lived abroad. Besides, my sister-in-law had been advised to have a Caesarean section as she is very petite and Kerem was a large baby. My brother had everything organised, and had booked her in to a private clinic. 'Just because you bake bread doesn't mean you should deliver John's bread in Brussels, does it?' I teased my father in return. 'Anyway, I haven't passed all my exams yet!'

Looking back, I'm surprised to recall that my training didn't affect how I felt about Nevim's pregnancy in any way. I didn't worry more than anyone else as we counted down the months and waited excitedly for news of Kerem's safe arrival. Nevim was my sister-in-law, not a patient, and despite tragic cases like Mrs Wainwright's, which still weighed heavily on my mind, for the most part I remained full of the optimism of youth. I had eagerly awaited this very exciting new arrival and I couldn't wait to meet him.

My mum had departed on the first available train and was planning to stay and help Nevim for three weeks while John went back to his job as a journalist for United Press International.

I was absolutely thrilled at becoming an auntie. Kerem was the first baby born into our family for many years. He would be loved and cherished, and I felt grateful that my brother and his wife had the means to give him the best possible start in life. If only every baby could be as lucky as Kerem.

Chapter Fourteen

'She's at top o' stairs!'

'There you are!' a familiar voice called out. 'Wherever did you get to, Linda?'

'Sorry, Mrs Tattersall,' I replied, 'Had to see Miss Sefton about my exam.'

'Yes, I'm sure you did, but Gwyneth Griffiths's baby won't know anything about that. Let's go. She got her husband to phone for us, and I must have had the message more than ten minutes gone!'

Mrs Tattersall carried a pager which she called a 'bleep' and when husbands and neighbours, and occasionally even the labouring mothers themselves, called from phone boxes on street corners, a message was relayed via the hospital switchboard operator, telling Mrs Tattersall she was needed. The majority of homes in the district had no telephone and, typically, the 'pips' went on the payphone before anything more detailed than the name of the patient and possibly an address were relayed to the telephonist. As a result Mrs Tattersall rarely had the opportunity to make any sort of assessment of the situation before she dashed off to what might be a false alarm or an imminent delivery. This meant she had to treat each call as if it might be an emergency, which accounted for her always appearing to be in a tearing hurry.

I had grown used to my heart rate quickening whenever Mrs Tattersall used the word 'bleep', and that morning I responded as she had taught me to, immediately focusing on the job in hand. I took the gas and air cylinder from her and we dashed to the car park together, with me apologising again and having a job keeping up with her impressively fast pace.

'Don't worry, love,' Mrs Tattersall wheezed, hauling her heavy bag of equipment into the boot of the car. 'First baby, should be slow, and it's very close by. Had a couple of false alarms already, so we might be on a wasted journey in any case.'

It was November now and I'd been working alongside Mrs Tattersall for five months – long enough to know she often said something along those lines. Even if her own heart was pounding faster and faster as we sped to each labouring mother, you would never have known it.

'I remember Mrs Griffiths,' I said, registering that she lived close to Moira Petty along Hope Street. 'Little two-up, two-down, isn't it?'

'Yes, one of them you can't swing a cat in,' Mrs Tattersall sighed. She paused for a moment to light a cigarette before pushing her foot hard on the accelerator.

Mr Griffiths threw the front door open dramatically as we stepped out of the trusty Avenger less than ten minutes later.

'Midwife's here!' he called to his wife upstairs. He turned back to us. 'Come quick, baby's coming!' he told me, his voice agitated, imploring me to get a move on. With mounting panic in his voice, he added breathlessly, 'She's at top o' stairs!'

There was a narrow hallway at the foot of the stairs and when I stepped inside and looked up I was greeted by the startling sight of Mrs Griffiths standing on the very top step, groaning and holding two rather tatty-looking tartan tea towels between her legs. She was wearing a long skirt that was hitched up around her hips and I was shocked to see that she was, in fact, trying to hold the baby back in with the tea towels.

'I'll get the gear,' I heard Mrs Tattersall call over my shoulder as I shot up the stairs like a rat up a drainpipe.

'Don't worry, Mrs Griffiths,' I soothed. 'Let's get you comfortable.'

There was no way in the world I could have shifted her, so I helped Mrs Griffiths lie down right where she stood, on the tiny square of landing that divided the two bedrooms on either side of the house. She was a large woman and she filled the entire space, while I crouched perilously on the top stair.

'Waters went,' she gasped. 'Tried to stop baby comin' as best as I could.'

'Keep breathing and try not to push just yet,' I instructed. 'Mrs Tattersall is …'

'Right here!' I heard my mentor puff.

I turned and saw her mounting the stairs two at a time, gas and air in one hand and her equipment bag in the other. The sight of her instantly reassured me. I even managed a smile, as I saw that she still had her cigarette in her mouth as she dashed towards us. With no free hand, she was dragging on it through puckered lips.

Dropping her baggage, Mrs Tattersall deftly manoeuvred herself into a position behind Mrs Griffiths and rasped through her half-smoked cigarette: 'Try to squat, that's it, lean back on me, on my legs if you like … Linda, can you see the head?'

'Yes I can,' I answered, though I could barely see Mrs Tattersall through the swirls of grey smoke gathering all around us.

'It's coming!' Mrs Griffiths coughed.

Her baby daughter was born moments later into a thick cloud of smoke while Mrs Tattersall continued to suck on the last dregs of her cigarette. The elated parents didn't seem to bother about that one bit, and I had long ago learned never to be surprised by what happened on my rounds with Mrs Tattersall.

Mr Griffiths, who was standing at the bottom of the stairs, gave us a hearty round of applause when he heard the little girl cry, while Mrs Griffiths thanked us over and over again and apologised for leaving it so late to phone.

'Good job I had the tea towels,' she said. 'I didn't want the baby to arrive before you did. Anyway, I can't thank you enough, I really can't.'

As I drove home from work on my moped that evening I was mulling over the events of the day and feeling quietly pleased with myself for dealing with Mrs Griffiths so calmly in the circumstances. It was very dark, damp and foggy. My legs were aching with tiredness as I rode the moped, but my mind was alert with the excitement of the day. I was almost a qualified midwife and I was thoroughly enjoying myself, delivering babies out in the community. I'd been studying hard, too, and I was fairly confident I would pass my final exam, which was an oral and written test, without a hitch.

I'd heard there was a woman expecting triplets attending the antenatal clinic, and I thought about how interesting it would be to be involved in their birth next year. Perhaps I could ask if that were possible? Of course it was possible, I realised, thrillingly. I was already capable of delivering babies all by myself, and I would be a fully fledged, qualified midwife by then, I was sure. I had delivered Lorinda Louise and little Jimmy, and I had all but delivered Mrs Griffiths's baby today in such unconventional conditions. What a triumph!

As I approached the last set of traffic lights before home I became aware that the red Hillman Imp in the left-hand lane beside me was drifting across the white line on the road. Blinking through the drizzle I decided to speed up to get past the little car as quickly as possible. I accelerated, and a terrifying noise filled my ears. I couldn't make it out. It was the crunch of metal on metal. It was the eerie screech of brakes not working fast enough. It was the sound of me yelling and crying out, becoming painfully aware that I was lying on the pavement on the opposite side of the wet road to where my moped lay.

Mr Fox was the motorist's name. He took me home, shaking uncontrollably, in his damaged car and told Graham what had happened.

'She hit the side of me and went straight over the bonnet,' I heard him explain, white as a sheet. 'I'm very sorry, I didn't see her. I don't think it was anybody's fault. Poor visibility. Wet road, I'm afraid.' I had to agree with him, though I wasn't sure exactly how the accident happened.

Remarkably, my coat and uniform were unscathed. I had a large, throbbing bruise on my hip but no cuts or even scratches despite this being a far worse crash than my accident at the doors of Casualty. I sat shaking from head to foot and nursing a cup of sweet tea while Graham gave Mr Fox five pounds to cover the damage to his dented car and took the details of where my moped needed to be picked up from. It was propped up next to a lamppost on the side of the road, and would probably need a bit of work done to it, Mr Fox advised. I'm pretty sure he caused the accident, but I can't be certain I didn't steer into him in the heat of the moment when I accelerated, and I was happy for Graham to give him the money.

'I think it's time we thought about getting you a car,' Graham said.

I nodded half-heartedly. The accident had really frightened me and in that moment the last thing I wanted to think about was taking to the roads again, especially in a car, but I didn't want Graham to worry.

'The girls at work said it's easy to pass your driving test when you're a nurse,' I told him, giving a brave little laugh.

'How come?' Graham asked curiously.

'Apparently the trick is to wear your nurse's uniform and hitch your skirt up an inch or two,' I smiled. 'They say it works every time, even if you're not much good behind the wheel.'

Graham laughed, which is what I wanted him to do. I was feeling embarrassed about the crash, and now the initial shock had subsided I wanted to play down how much it had shaken me up. In my job I was used to being the one people looked to for help, not the other way around. I joined in with Graham's laughter, even though it made my sore body ache.

'Put your feet up, Linda, while I go and get the moped. We'll fix it up and sell it and get you a decent car.'

Once I was qualified my pay would increase and we would comfortably be able to afford a new car. It seemed like a good idea.

As soon as Graham had gone I shuffled tentatively into the kitchen. Over the previous few weeks I'd made two Christmas cakes, one for my parents and one for my in-laws. I'd followed an old recipe I had on a typed card from school, when we'd been taught traditional baking in Domestic Science. I really wanted these Christmas cakes to be perfect. Both sets of parents had given us so much support in our first year of marriage, and I wanted to prove that I was the perfect little wife, capable of running the home as well as working hard for my final exam and completing Part Two of my training.

The day before, I'd put the finishing touches to the marzipan and royal icing, and now, even though my hands were still trembling and sore, I added the finishing touch – a red and green frill around each cake – and set them on top of the fridge for safe-keeping. They were loaded with dried fruit and brandy and weighed an absolute ton, and my arms ached just lifting them.

Graham returned just as I put them down. 'I'll get the dinner on,' I called down the hallway. 'I feel as right as rain now.'

'More than can be said about your moped,' he remarked.

The Honda needed quite a bit of patching up, but Graham said he would deal with it, and then place an advert in the *Manchester Evening News* to sell it as soon as I had passed my driving test.

'Mind that paint in the vestibule,' I shouted, suddenly remembering I'd left two tins of emulsion balanced next to the telephone table. I wanted to spruce up the paintwork in the lounge before Christmas, so determined was I to prove my worth as a competent little homemaker.

December 1970 was an incredibly busy month. The wards were teeming with patients and I found myself working long hours and, as I was still a pupil midwife, being given the worst 'off-duty'. This meant moving around the wards frequently and taking on more night shifts, which was extremely tiring.

One evening I arrived at work feeling utterly exhausted before I'd even started. I'd spent the day cleaning the house in preparation for the decorating, as well as writing out scores of Christmas cards. Graham and I had been receiving cards for a week or so now, but I had scarcely had time to put pen to paper. The arrival of a card from Linda Mochri had jolted me into action. 'All fine here in bonny Scotland,' she had written brightly. 'Hope you are well.'

I realised, to my shame, that the best part of a year had passed since I'd heard from Linda and I had no idea how she was getting on. I had been so caught up in my own life I had not made time to keep in touch with old friends. I hadn't a clue how Nessa, Anne or Jo were doing either, and I resolved to send them all a Christmas card and wish them well for 1971. In my heart I knew that our friendship, as we knew it, could never be rekindled, but nevertheless I hoped to keep in contact.

'You look shattered!' Barbara Lees remarked when she saw me putting on my apron on the postnatal ward that night. 'And it's not a good night to be tired!'

'Why ever not?' I asked.

'The wards are absolutely fit to burst. I heard they had two women labouring in the same delivery room earlier and had to wheel one of them out while the other gave birth!'

'No! Why is it so busy?'

'No idea, but thank goodness we're getting a new hospital, that's all I can say.'

I nodded. There had been a lot of excited talk about the new maternity unit. Our old maternity facilities within Ashton General would be gradually shut down, and by the end of 1971 we would have a large, purpose-built maternity unit, which was being built next to the existing hospital.

With more women than ever opting to have a hospital birth as opposed to a home delivery, it was anticipated the new maternity unit would be an extremely popular and thriving facility.

Talking to Barbara, I suddenly had a sense of being in the right place at the right time, which spurred me on that night despite my weariness. That feeling was magnified when I was summoned to see Miss Sefton before I began my duties. I had a good idea what she wanted to talk about, and I had been waiting for this moment. My record of deliveries had been sent to the Central Midwives Board for scrutiny, and I had been awaiting the result of my final exam, which I thought had gone very well. I had been hoping that any day now Miss Sefton would be able to confirm that I had passed my Part Two. This was it!

'Congratulations,' she said warmly when I entered her office. She expressed her great pleasure in informing me that I had passed my final exam with flying colours and that I had ably assisted in the various required births from March to December. Margaret Mulligan had been right, I thought. It wasn't that hard to clock up the necessary deliveries.

'In passing Part Two you have automatically earned yourself a position as a staff midwife here at Ashton General Hospital,' Miss Sefton confirmed. 'In my opinion you should stay here, as you will probably be ready for a sister's post in twelve months' time.'

This news was delivered without fuss, though I was given a fancy certificate that informed me I was now entitled to inclusion in the Midwives Roll. It also declared that I, Linda Mary Buckley, was authorised to 'hold herself out as certified' under the Midwives Act of 1951. I was a qualified midwife at last! What an achievement!

I knew that staff midwives automatically qualified for a sister's post after twelve months on the job, although of course you only got the job if there was a vacancy. With the new maternity unit opening, there would be plenty of sisters' posts to fill, which was extremely good timing for me.

I rushed out of Miss Sefton's office feeling fantastic. This was a very significant moment for me, and it felt very special. I had been a student for more than four years, all told, and this day was a real landmark. I felt truly ecstatic.

I could dedicate my whole life to delivering babies now. It was what I was meant to do, I was sure of it. Being a nursery nurse might have been a feasible alternative, but it wouldn't have been the perfect job for me. I was meant to be a midwife. That's how I felt, very powerfully now. I had achieved my dream thus far and I was certain I would never stop fizzing with pride whenever I heard those words, 'The midwife's here!'

Back on the busy ward there was no time for further reflection, and my first task that night was to assist two new mothers with breastfeeding.

'Linda, see to those two in beds three and four, will ya?' Sister Kelly ordered, scratching her bosom earnestly. 'They've decided to try breastfeeding, so they have, but aren't making a very good job of it if the truth be told. Poor little mites'll be starvin', the way they're goin' on.'

She rolled her eyes and sucked on her teeth as I headed off to meet Audrey Asprey and Eileen Yates, who had given birth to their respective daughters Adele and Donna within an hour of each other. Both women were bright-eyed and in their early twenties, and they explained to me enthusiastically that they'd heard a radio programme about the benefits of breastfeeding and wanted to give it a try, to give their daughters the 'best possible start in life'.

'Good for you,' I complimented them. 'We don't get too many mums wanting to breastfeed, even though as midwives we're taught to encourage it. After all, breast milk is the perfect food for baby, and is always at the right temperature.'

They both looked very pleased with themselves and listened attentively as I discussed the basic principles of breastfeeding and described how they needed to try to relax in order to get the baby to 'latch on' to the nipple correctly.

'I'll be back over in a little while, after the bottles are dished out,' I said.

An hour passed and my feet and head were throbbing. I'd prepared all the bottles in the steaming milk kitchen and changed three or four babies in the nursery, including Adele and Donna. Betty, one of the hard-working auxiliaries, returned the babies to their mothers while I dished out bottles of milk before going to help with the breastfeeding.

To my delight, when I arrived at Audrey's bedside she was already breastfeeding beautifully, the little girl at her breast guzzling milk greedily and contentedly.

'I don't think you need any help at all,' I smiled. 'Well done! You've got that down to a fine art!'

Just at that moment, I heard a worried little voice from the other side of the curtain around Audrey's bed. 'Excuse me, Nurse, can you come here a minute?'

I stepped out through the curtain to find Eileen standing before me with a confused look in her eyes.

'What's the matter?' I asked.

Eileen hesitated for a moment before hissing in my ear, 'The thing is, Nurse, Adele is in the nursery and Donna isn't, and I think ...'

'Whatever do you mean?' I asked, my heart rate quickening as my brain caught up with what she was saying.

'Audrey is feeding Donna!' Eileen exclaimed loudly.

I pulled back the curtain to reveal the well-fed baby in Audrey's arms giving a contented burp as she nestled on her chest.

'Bloody hell!' Audrey yelped, handing Donna over to her mother as if she were a hot potato. 'Does that mean I've got to start all over again with Adele? I'm not sure I've got any milk left!'

'I'll fetch Adele right away,' I said, dashing off swiftly. I'd never known Betty to make a single mistake before, let alone one of this magnitude. Normally the auxiliaries were marvellous and a crucial part of the team. Midwives treasured them as they were always there when you needed them, not only fetching and carrying but acting as another pair of eyes and ears. Betty must have been run off her feet today, I thought.

I returned from the nursery to find the two women chuckling merrily away. 'There's no need to apologise,' Eileen was saying. 'I'm just glad my Donna's had a good feed – first proper stuff she's had!'

With incredible good nature and impressive ease, Eileen later went on to breastfeed the real Adele, and as far as the women were concerned that was the end of it. They wouldn't hear a word of apology and both said how uncanny it was that their daughters had been born so close together, and how alike the two little girls looked, especially in their matching hospital gowns. Neither woman blamed the auxiliary, despite the fact both babies wore name tags and were in labelled cots.

Looking back, I marvel at how times have changed. If that were to happen today, blood tests would definitely be called for, and most probably lawyers too. But this was a time when HIV was unheard of in maternity units and litigation was a word you rarely heard, so life carried on with no harm done.

I reported the matter to the night sister, of course, but I am pleased to say I heard no mention of the mix-up ever again. Nevertheless, my nerves were shot to pieces at the end of my shift and I couldn't wait to get home and unwind.

As I was leaving the hospital at 7 a.m. the next morning I ran into Mrs Tattersall, who was rushing to a home birth.

'Fancy coming with me?' she asked. 'Sixth baby, would you believe. Should be quick, up on the Moss. Husband makes a very good brew.'

'Do you mind if I don't?' I said politely. 'I think I need to get some sleep. I've had quite an eventful shift.'

Intuitive as ever, Mrs Tattersall knew I had a tale to tell and urged me to do so. I was so tired I could hardly relate the story without getting Adele mixed up with Donna and Eileen confused with Audrey all over again.

Mrs Tattersall laughed like a drain. 'It happens, Linda love,' she said. 'All's well that ends well, that's what I say.' She put her hand on my shoulder, and I sensed she had a tale to tell too.

'A lot worse things can happen, Linda. Perhaps this is not the best time to tell you, but then again I don't know when it ever is. I heard some sad news last night. Moira Petty's little boy, Jimmy, has died. He had a serious heart defect. Nothing could be done for him, poor soul.'

I felt my legs buckle beneath me, I was so shocked and upset. I could picture poor Moira, labouring in the cold and damp in that front parlour, and I remembered how pleased I had been to see her little boy dressed up in his brand new clothes despite the poverty he was born into. I had hoped his life could be better than his mother's, but now he had no life at all.

'That's awful,' I gasped. 'That's just awful.'

'Well,' Mrs Tattersall replied thoughtfully, 'it might have been a blessing. The poor little lad had enough disadvantages in life. A heart defect was perhaps one too many to bear.'

I knew what she meant but it didn't make me feel any less sad about his passing.

When I arrived home, I fell through the front door feeling as if I'd been put through a wringer and was greeted unexpectedly by Sue, our Red Setter. Normally she was asleep in her basket at this early hour, but she jumped up on me excitedly, taking me completely by surprise.

There was something white all around her mouth, and when I looked closely and took a sniff I realised to my dismay that it was icing – or the royal icing from my Christmas cakes, to be precise.

'Sue!' I hissed. She bounded off and I went to give chase but tripped clumsily over something hard in the hallway. It was one of the tins of white emulsion paint I'd left standing there, ready for the decorating. It overturned and spilled all over the hall carpet, making me burst into tears on the spot. Sue barked loudly, and I followed her through to the kitchen to find both of my lovingly baked Christmas cakes half-eaten on the floor. I sat on the cold tiles beside the crumbs and mess and sobbed into my hands.

Graham appeared at the kitchen door.

'Whatever's going on?' he asked, rubbing sleep from his eyes and looking bemused.

'Nothing,' I shrugged, wiping away my tears. 'Just a day in the life of a midwife, I suppose.'

He put his arm around me. 'There's no need to cry about spilt paint, you know ...'

'I'm not,' I replied. Poor little Jimmy was dead. As if I would waste my tears crying about a ruined carpet! 'And I don't care about the cakes either, not really,' I sniffed.

'So what is it?' Graham asked.

'Just work. It's hard sometimes. And sometimes you have to sit down and have a good cry. This is one of those moments. It comes with the job. I'll be all right in a bit. You go back to bed.'

I found myself saying a similar thing to him when I returned home from my shift on Christmas Day 1970. While the rest of the family tucked in to cold turkey sandwiches in the evening I could think of nothing but what had happened at work earlier that day, but it wasn't fair to burden Graham.

'How was it?' Graham asked brightly, fetching me a Babycham. 'Any Christmas Day babies?'

'Yes,' I replied warily. 'Six today. Hard day, but I'll be all right in a bit. Let me just get changed.'

I went upstairs alone and thought about the babies born that day. I had delivered two of them, and they were absolutely beautiful. One was a bouncing ten-pound boy named Nicholas who was so chubby he looked as though he had elastic bands around his wrists and ankles, and the other was a dainty girl named Angela, who was just under six pounds.

Their respective parents were ecstatic, and I experienced a rush of pure joy as I handed each mother her child for that first momentous cuddle. Both babies felt extra-special, being born on Christmas Day, and I felt incredibly honoured to have brought such wonderful little miracles into the world.

'This is why I do the job,' I thought to myself as I surveyed the postnatal ward later, and met some of the other precious newborns delivered that day. I usually went to visit my ladies before I finished my shift, to check they were all right. It's not an obligatory part of the job, of course, but it's something I have always enjoyed doing.

We had a lot of fun on the wards that day, I recall. Some of the midwives played tricks on the patients, making what we called 'apple-pie beds' by turning the top sheet back on itself under the covers to make it impossible to get in without ending up in a proper muddle. One brave midwife also put KY Jelly on the telephones in the consultants' and sisters' offices, so each time they answered a call the handset slipped clean out of their grasp. It was all taken in good humour and there was a warm buzz around the hospital, which was decked out with tinsel and fairy lights.

Now, sitting alone upstairs in our bedroom at home, I reflected sadly on how the shine had been abruptly stripped from the day as I was finishing my shift and breezily wishing my colleagues a good evening.

'Hope you have a few more Christmas babies!' I smiled merrily.

'Well, things can only get better,' another midwife replied, ominously.

'What's happened?' I asked.

'Oh, Linda,' she said apologetically, 'I thought everyone must have heard. I shouldn't have mentioned it; it was careless of me. You go home, go and enjoy the rest of your day.'

'No, what have I missed?' I asked. 'You have to tell me now.'

My colleague sighed heavily and I saw that she was blinking back tears. 'There was a poor young girl brought in earlier, probably while you were occupied with Mrs Burrows and baby Angela. She was only sixteen and had her baby alone at home this morning. Very sadly, the baby died. Such a tragic case, today of all days.'

'Who was she?' I asked, shocked. 'Have I seen her in antenatal?'

'No,' came the reply. 'She is still at school and had hidden her pregnancy from everyone, so it appears. She had the baby in the toilet upstairs while her family ate Christmas dinner. The first they knew about it was when they heard her screams.'

This was such a sad story that I couldn't stop thinking about it all the way home. I couldn't begin to imagine what that poor girl had gone through, frightened and alone and in so much pain. It made my spirits sink completely, and I had to tell myself to count my lucky stars. I had a loving husband waiting for me in our warm and welcoming house, where there were no secrets and lies. Thinking about that poor girl made me cherish what I had so much more. I had a good life, and I wished others could be as fortunate as me.

'So six babies born today I hear, Linda!' my mother-in-law, Edith, beamed when I reappeared in the living room, glad to be free of my uniform at last. 'Well I never!'

I nodded and said no more. Sometimes, I thought, that was the best thing to do. Sometimes it was simply not the right time to talk about my job, and this was most definitely one of those moments. I certainly didn't want any of my loved ones to have their day spoilt too.

'I'm glad I haven't missed *Morecambe and Wise*,' I said brightly, biting into a peanut cracknel from a tin of Quality Street. I turned to the television as the comedy duo launched into their silly signature tune, 'Bring Me Sunshine'. The lyrics made me smile. 'In this world where we live, there should be more happiness/So much joy you can give, to each brand new bright tomorrow.' How very true, I mused to myself. Tomorrow is another day, and just think how many new babies will be born, lighting up their parents' worlds.

Chapter Fifteen

'He's not touching her privates!'

'Hey, Linda, fancy coming for a peep next door?'

It was Maggie, friendly as ever, and she was gesturing towards our new maternity unit that was being built tantalisingly close to the old facilities.

'Are we allowed?' I asked cautiously, knowing that the men who worked on the site wore hard hats and had cordoned off the entrance doors with thick sheeting.

'Barbara and I had a little look last week and nobody complained. Come on, it's exciting!'

Maggie ran off down the corridor with me in hot pursuit, and minutes later we had crossed the grounds and entered what was to be our bright new workplace, still very much under construction.

I blinked as I stepped inside the building, dazzled by the shiny newness of everything around me. The pure white walls were spotlessly clean and huge windows let light flood through the corridors, making everything glint. Even the smell was novel, with a potent mixture of fresh paint and plastic packaging hanging in the air. I felt prickles of excitement in my fingertips, and wanted to explore every nook and cranny of this fantastic new environment, which felt like a giant present we'd been given.

'Look, Linda,' Maggie gestured, pulling back a dustsheet that covered a ward doorway and letting me peer inside. 'These are going to be four-bedded wards. The windows over there will have brand-new Venetian blinds and they're to be double glazed, no less.'

The wards looked nothing like the old Nightingale wards I was used to. Tiptoeing around, I saw brochures showing fancy floral curtains that would be hung around the beds, brand new plastic washbowls and pictures of tooth mugs without a stain or a chip in sight. Maggie pointed out spacious rooms that would become state-of-the-art day rooms and nurseries, and there was even a flower bay, she exclaimed gleefully.

'I can't wait to start work in here,' I smiled.

'Nor can I!' Maggie replied. 'Come on, let's get back before Miss Sefton finds out what we're up to.'

We skipped back, giggling like a pair of schoolgirls.

'We're getting this whole unit all to ourselves, all five floors of it!' Maggie whooped. 'I can't believe it!'

From that day on I found myself counting down the months until we moved in. The date for the grand opening was set for 3 December 1971. That was ten months away, and I simply couldn't wait.

For the time being I was on the antenatal clinic in the old hospital, and I enjoyed telling the patients all about the imminent new facilities.

'What are you tellin' me for?' they joked. 'This is my last baby. I'll not be back after this one, mark my words!'

'That's what they all say,' I often replied. 'We'll see!'

One morning I was delighted to see Mrs Sully waiting for her antenatal check-up. She was one of my favourite ladies at that time, and I was very much hoping I would be lucky enough to deliver her first child, if I happened to be on duty when she went into labour. She was one of those women who positively glowed in pregnancy, to the point where it almost felt contagious.

'How are you feeling?' I asked as I took her blood pressure and listened to her baby's strong heartbeat through the Pinard trumpet I pressed to her abdomen.

'Flippin' fantastic!' she replied, which is what she always said.

Her cheeks were as pink as rosebuds and her dark brown hair seemed to get shinier on every visit as she bloomed and blossomed. I always felt radiant myself after being in Mrs Sully's presence.

'Trust me to time it so I'll be having my first baby in here instead of the new place,' she chuckled. 'Still, hopefully I'll be over the road for the next one!'

'That's forward planning for you,' I smiled. 'Most women can't bear to think about another pregnancy before they've got this one over and done with first.'

'I know, but I've felt so fantastic being pregnant I can't help dreaming about the next. I've always wanted a hatful of kids, I have.'

Next on my clinic list that day was a thin, anxious young girl called Dorothy Dunn who had asked me on her previous visit if she could bring her husband along to this next appointment.

'He's a bit nervous about everything, and so am I,' she had admitted apologetically, wringing her bony fingers. 'I know you don't like having men in here, but I'd like it if he could hold my hand, see what's going on. I think it might be good for us both.'

'That's fine,' I had replied. 'It's not that we don't like having men in here; it's just not what most couples do.'

I thought about that other poor young man I'd seen unceremoniously pushed out of the doors of one of the very first antenatal clinics I worked on, but that was almost a year ago now, and I could see that things had very slowly started to change.

'It's not *quite* as unusual as it used to be to bring your husband in,' I continued, wanting to put Mrs Dunn at her ease. 'We're starting to see one or two husbands shuffling in from time to time, and they're very welcome in my opinion. If that's what you want, it's perfectly fine by me.'

I wondered if I might rue my words when I met Mr Dunn. He was a lanky, bespectacled young man with a miserable grey pallor. Like his wife, he was very young – probably barely out of his teens – and he appeared terribly nervous. I'd noticed that Mrs Dunn had bitten her fingernails to the quick, and now I saw that her husband had done the same. Mr Dunn looked worried sick and was fidgeting with his knitted tie and looking at the floor as he tentatively followed his twitchy wife into a side room.

'Please try to make yourself comfortable,' I implored, showing Mr Dunn to a chair beside the examination couch.

He sat in stony silence, looking like a condemned man, while I took his wife's blood pressure, weighed her and checked her ankles for signs of swelling. I got the impression he didn't want to be there at all.

'What a pretty wedding band,' I remarked to Mrs Dunn, trying to lighten the atmosphere as I listened to baby's heartbeat and palpated her abdomen to assess the size and position of her baby. 'Have you been married long?'

'Eight months,' she replied shyly. 'I caught very quickly, on honeymoon in Anglesey.'

Mr Dunn blushed to the roots of his mousy hairline and continued to stare at the floor, no doubt wishing it would swallow him up.

I smiled. 'The doctor would like to carry out an internal examination, to check everything is as it should be.' This wasn't a task midwives performed at the antenatal clinic in those days. 'Mr Dunn, you are welcome to stay, or you can step outside if you wish.'

'I'll stay,' he muttered, keeping his eyes fixed on his shoes.

I was surprised by this response. Of the very few men who accompanied their wives to antenatal check-ups, I couldn't recall a single one who stayed in the room while a vaginal examination was carried out. Mr Dunn had agreed he would accompany his wife, however, and he was clearly a man of his word.

I asked Mrs Dunn to remove her pants, and the doctor arrived seconds later and swiftly began his examination.

'What is he doing?' Mr Dunn demanded hotly, pointing at the startled doctor but addressing his question to me. He jumped out of his seat as if his backside had been set alight. 'Why is he touching my wife there?'

I was so taken aback at his unexpected outburst I was rendered speechless for a moment. My eyes darted between Mr and Mrs Dunn and the doctor, who gave me a look as if to say, 'Deal with it, will you?' and carried on.

I began to explain, as calmly as possible, that the doctor was simply carrying out a routine internal examination, to check that everything was in order in advance of the imminent birth.

'Not her privates!' Mr Dunn spluttered, incredulous. 'He's not touching her privates!'

Mrs Dunn looked mortified and bit her quivering lips while the doctor finished his examination and stepped swiftly away, giving me the nod that his work was done. I thought the poor girl might cry.

'I'm sorry,' I said gently to Mr Dunn as the doctor scribbled up his notes and sped out of the room. 'But it's our duty to …'

'Why?' Mr Dunn demanded. He appeared totally flummoxed.

'Well, when the baby arrives, of course it travels down the birth canal, which is in fact the vagina,' I said, slowly cottoning on to the astonishing fact that Mr Dunn had no idea how babies were delivered.

'Not from her privates!' he gasped in horror.

'Er, yes, the baby comes from her privates.'

Mr Dunn's forehead was shiny with sweat as he glanced from one to the other of us, then said 'Excuse me' and hurried out of the room. It was left to Mrs Dunn to say exactly what I was thinking.

'Where on earth does he think babies come from?' she gaped, open-mouthed.

'He knows now, and that's what matters,' I said as tactfully as possible. 'I think it was a happy accident you brought him in today. I can't imagine what might have happened if he hadn't figured it out before the birth.'

'I thought it was a good idea,' Mrs Dunn replied. 'I wasn't sure how much he understood … or how little.'

I told my friend Marjorie that story one night during a drinks party at our house, taking care not to reveal the identity of the hapless father-to-be in case he was one of her customers at the bank.

'I still can't get over it,' I told her. 'I know most men don't have anything to do with childbirth, but how can anyone be so naïve?'

'It beggars belief,' Marjorie agreed. 'Did he think the stork was going to deliver his baby, or what?'

'I have absolutely no idea,' I said. 'We'll never know, but one thing's for sure, I'll never forget that young man!'

It was Easter 1971 when I met my new nephew, Kerem, for the very first time. John and Nevim brought him over to England when he was about six months old, and I was delighted to see them all at my parents' house after work one evening.

'He's huge!' I exclaimed when I saw the chunky bundle in my mum's arms, draining a bottle of milk like there was no tomorrow.

'He's absolutely perfect, just right for his age,' Mum clucked. 'You're just so used to dealing with newborns, Linda.'

She was right. To me, a typical baby weighed about seven or eight pounds, had to be encouraged to take milk and looked and felt incredibly fragile. By contrast, Kerem was a very sturdy little boy indeed.

I held him in my arms and fell in love with him instantly. The shine in his eyes, the sweet smell of his tufty fair hair and the musical gurgles that bubbled from his little lips made my heart swell. He was adorable, and I was totally smitten.

'Look at you,' Nevim grinned. 'It's as if you have never held a baby before!'

'I haven't held one like this before, not one of ours,' I replied.

Kerem began to grizzle and I suggested he might need another bottle, as I'd noticed how rapidly he demolished the last one.

'Our midwife told me just to give him two ounces at a time, then stop for a while and burp him,' Nevim explained.

'Oh,' I replied, thinking that if he were one of my babies at the hospital I'd keep feeding him if he'd take more. I held my tongue, though, aware that I was here in the role of auntie, not midwife. 'You know best, Nevim.'

Mum and I exchanged knowing glances, and I realised we were both sharing the same thought about a universal truth: brand new mothers are all the same. Fired up with powerful maternal instincts, they all hang on their midwife's every word, never daring to deviate from the professional's advice lest they put their new baby's life in peril.

As an experienced mother, Mum knew that this phase would pass and Nevim would make her own rules when she was good and ready. I knew this too, despite being the only childless woman in the room. It was quite a strange experience, and of course I couldn't help wondering what I would be like as a mother one day, given my job. I wasn't quite ready yet, I knew that. I was too involved in laying the foundations of my career and I had only just turned twenty-three years of age, so time was still on my side. But looking at Kerem, I knew more than ever that I definitely wanted to have babies of my own before too long.

John and my father struck up a conversation about decimalisation, which had taken place just a couple of months earlier and was still a hot topic for debate.

'How are your customers coping?' John asked Dad. 'I can't imagine the older generation taking too kindly to the change, if you'll pardon the pun!'

'Let's just say that if I had half a crown for every time I've heard a customer ask, "How much is that in old money?" I'd be a rich man,' Dad chortled.

Mum chipped in with a funny story about old Mrs Woodcock, one of Lawton's Confectioners' most loyal customers.

'She's been chuntering on about the loss of her beloved shillings and sixpences for yonks,' Mum said. 'I kept telling her that by the time Decimal Day finally came, she'd be well prepared. It's been long enough coming, what with all those adverts on the television telling us the same thing over and over again. But do you know what she said to me yesterday when I tried to explain it all for the umpteenth time?'

We all shook our heads and waited for the punchline. 'Without a word of a lie, Mrs Woodcock said to me: "I still don't understand, I'm afraid, Mrs Lawton, but don't you worry yourself. I'm going to live in Southport with my daughter, and they don't do it there."'

'Mrs Sully is in the first-stage room,' Barbara Lees told me when I arrived for a shift on the labour ward several weeks later, on a balmy morning in May 1971.

'Oh, that's good,' I smiled at Barbara, who was now a sister. 'I was hoping I'd be on duty when she came in. She's one of those ladies who always brightens up my day.'

Mrs Sully was propped up comfortably on a chair next to the bed in the labour room. She looked as radiant as ever and greeted me with a wide grin.

'I hoped I'd be seeing you this week,' I told her. 'How are you getting on?'

'Marvellous!' she said. 'Hurts with contractions, but they're regular enough and I'm doing all right with the pain, touch wood.'

She leaned over and touched the wooden trim on a cupboard.

'That's good,' I said. 'Can I ask you to pop in the toilet and provide me with a urine sample, then I'll take a look and see how things are progressing?'

'No bother!' she smiled, easing herself out of her chair and padding her way slowly across to the bathroom, clutching her stomach protectively.

I checked Mrs Sully's notes while she was gone, and waited a minute. She was taking longer than expected, and I was just about to call through to see if she needed any assistance when the toilet door swung open abruptly, startling me.

'There's something between my legs,' Mrs Sully announced, her voice quivering.

'Let's have a look, shall we?' I said calmly, though my heart-beat had quickened considerably.

I registered her demeanour. Mrs Sully looked flustered but was standing perfectly upright, breathing deeply but regularly. She was wearing a long gypsy skirt with tiny mirrored sequins on it, which she was hitching up at the front with one hand, and her knickers were round her knees. There was no way she'd had the baby as there simply hadn't been time, thank goodness, and she didn't even appear to be in the advanced stages of labour.

'Let's get you up on the bed,' I said, steering her slowly across the room, 'and we'll see what's going on.'

My heart skipped a beat when I lifted her skirt but I tried not to let the shock show in my face. Part of the umbilical cord was hanging between her legs and I immediately remembered the words of Miss Greeves, one of the tutors during my training.

'This is known as cord prolapse and is an emergency situation,' Miss Greeves had told us during a lecture, showing us an alarming diagram.

I remembered getting goosebumps all over when she first described this life-threatening scenario, and I got them again now, tenfold.

'The baby's head presses on the cord and you have to literally hold the head back inside the vagina so it doesn't compress the cord and cut off the oxygen supply. You also need to keep the cord as warm as possible. An emergency Caesarean is the only way to deliver the baby safely, and it must be performed as swiftly as possible.'

I went into autopilot, the words 'swiftly as possible' crashing round my head. I pressed the red emergency buzzer on the wall to summon Sister Lees, tipped the foot of Mrs Sully's bed up to relieve some of the pressure of gravity pushing down on the baby, and pushed my fingers inside her to tuck the cord back in as best I could to keep it warm, while at the same time holding the baby's head so it didn't descend any further and crush the cord.

'Try to stay as calm as possible,' I told Mrs Sully, my throat as dry as an old bone. 'It's best for the baby. Help is on the way.'

Mrs Sully began to cry a bit but, mercifully, didn't ask any questions. 'My husband is at work,' was all she said. 'He won't be here for another hour or so.'

Seconds later Sister Lees appeared, took one swift look and said, 'I'll alert the duty doctor and theatre.'

All the colour had drained from Mrs Sully's face now and she was shaking her head and saying, 'Please tell me everything will be all right'.

'We're doing the best we can,' I reassured her as two theatre technicians raced in and prepared to push Mrs Sully's bed to the operating theatre. 'We'll get you to theatre as quickly as we can, then we'll have to deliver your baby by Caesarean section.'

I was desperately trying to keep my fingers off the cord and on the baby's head inside the birth canal. It was incredibly awkward, especially as the bed had to be raised onto its wheels before being pushed rapidly down the corridor. As we sped around a corner I almost lost my grip on the baby's head and I decided there was only one thing for it; with a tremendous leap, I launched myself onto the moving bed beside Mrs Sully so I could hold my fingers in the best position to keep the baby safe. I thanked my lucky stars I was still a nimble size eight and able to squeeze onto the slim patch of mattress beside her left thigh.

'You're doing ever so well. Just try to stay calm.'

From this position I managed to keep my fingers in place as Mrs Sully was carefully but swiftly lifted off the bed and placed on a theatre table. I felt relieved that I had done exactly what was required in the circumstances and everything had gone to plan, so far. Mrs Sully was silent, breathing deeply, and looked utterly terrified.

'Can you feel the cord pulsating?' the surgeon asked me.

'Yes,' I replied positively. 'Yes I can.'

Gregory, the anaesthetist, got to work immediately. I noted that less than ten minutes had elapsed since Mrs Sully's trip to the toilet, which meant we had every chance of delivering her baby safely by Caesarean. All we had to do was anaesthetise her as quickly as possible while continuing to keep the cord warm, pulsating and uncrushed by the baby's head.

Gregory placed an oxygen mask over Mrs Sully's nose and mouth to help improve the baby's oxygen supply, and he administered an intravenous drug to anaesthetise her.

Any moment now, I thought, she'll be unconscious and the surgeon can make the incision in her abdomen. This might be a tricky Caesarean, with the baby already pushing down low, but we had every chance of success as we'd got her to theatre so rapidly.

To my horror, though, instead of falling into a deep sleep, Mrs Sully suddenly began thrashing and fighting on the theatre bed. This can happen when a patient is very tense and frightened, but I knew it could be catastrophic in these circumstances. I was still doing my best to simultaneously hold the baby's head back and protect the cord, but Mrs Sully was in such a state I was struggling to keep my fingers in the correct position inside her.

Minutes passed and the tension in the theatre was mounting. The surgeon surveyed his patient with alarm while an ashen-faced Gregory tried to inject her with more anaesthetic. Although her eyes were closed, unbelievably she continued to jerk and struggle on the table. I could feel the foetal heartbeat start to fade in the cord and it became apparent that we needed a miracle.

At last, several minutes later, Mrs Sully's body stopped moving. Thank God, she was finally fully unconscious, with a tube down her throat to keep her airways open. The relieved surgeon immediately got to work making an incision vertically down Mrs Sully's belly, while I prayed silently this precious baby would make it.

Another quick glance at the watch on my chest told me it had taken a full twenty minutes to anaesthetise Mrs Sully, and I felt tears prick my eyes. I couldn't see her face now as it was covered with a green theatre cloth. I was glad of that. I couldn't bear to look at her if things went wrong. I held my breath as the surgeon expertly opened her up and lifted a blood-smeared but perfectly formed little boy into the world.

The baby breathed when his cord was cut, but only just. He took gasping breaths, fighting for life, and I feared the worst. As I whisked him into a waiting resuscitaire for the paediatrician to take over, I knew his life was hanging in the balance. With the cord falling as it had, the baby's oxygen supply had been restricted for too long. I could feel sadness crushing my lungs as I watched the paediatrician working hard on the little mite, warming him, massaging him and willing him to live.

In the end Mrs Sully's son lived for just fifteen minutes. When the paediatrician shook his head and stepped away from the resuscitaire, the whole room fell deathly silent. I could hear my heartbeat thumping in my ears, too loud, too strong. This wasn't fair.

Had he survived, Mrs Sully's little boy may have been severely brain damaged because of the oxygen deprivation, but I knew that would be precious little comfort for his bereaved mother. There was nothing that could soften the blow of this dreadful loss. What could anybody say or do to make it less painful? Nothing, because nothing at all could bring her son back to life. Of all people, how could this have happened to sunny Mrs Sully? Until that day she had appeared not to have a care in the world. I couldn't get over it.

Later, when Mrs Sully came round and was alert enough to talk, I held her hand as I prepared myself to explain what had happened and answer her questions. In a case like this, the doctor would normally have spoken to her, but as I knew her from antenatal clinic it was right I should be the one who was there for her, with a doctor on standby in case he was needed.

Before either of us spoke Mrs Sully burst into tears. 'I know it's not good, Nurse,' she sobbed. 'I know my baby is dead, I know it.'

My eyes were full of tears as I bent over the bed and hugged her. 'I'm so sorry. You had a little boy. The doctors did everything they possibly could. Sometimes that is just not enough.'

The baby had already been taken away, and I had never seen a woman look so utterly bereft as Mrs Sully did that day. The roses I was used to seeing in her cheeks had disappeared, leaving a ghostly paleness in their place.

Before she was discharged, I knew Mrs Sully would need to be given post-operative advice about her Caesarean scar, and I thought what an awful task that would be for another midwife. Normally women joked that they'd be glad of the rest when we told them not to hang out washing or get down on their hands and knees and mop the kitchen floor for six weeks. They generally weren't worried that they'd undergone major surgery and would have a scar to prove it for the rest of their lives, because they had a beautiful new baby in return.

I knew there would be no jokes with Mrs Sully. Luck had deserted her when she needed it most, and there was nothing anyone could say or do to put things right. I wrote up her notes with a heavy heart that night, and at the end of my shift I took out an extra piece of paper and jotted down some personal notes, for myself.

It's been a terrible day. I want to write down my thoughts and feelings here and now. It's not fair to unload on Graham, but I need to get this out. What would Sister Mary Francis say about this? Can I still believe there is a God, and if so why does he let such dreadful things happen to such lovely people as Mrs Sully? There is no answer that can satisfy me. I know some people say these things happen to make us all stronger, to make us grow and make us better people. I'm finding it hard to accept, but I know I must. It's part of my job and I have to accept how cruel and powerful nature can be. I pray I can stay strong, because I want to carry on doing my job as well as I can. I hope Mrs Sully has another baby one day. She deserves some good fortune. Thinking of her with another child in her arms makes me feel better. I will hold that thought.

I tucked the note in my pocket and smiled wistfully. I remembered Sister Craddock once telling me at the MRI 'it's good to debrief', and I agreed with her wholeheartedly. I felt better for getting that off my chest, and I vowed always to try to take a minute or two to write down my feelings when I felt the need to unload.

I revisited that day in my head countless times over the following weeks and months. Mrs Sully still needed to have postnatal visits, even without a baby, and each time I saw her name on the community midwife's list I pictured her grief-stricken face and wanted to cry all over again. I rarely let the tears fall, though. Instead, I made myself imagine Mrs Sully coming back into the antenatal clinic with a brand new bump and fresh roses in her cheeks. 'I've always wanted a hatful of kids, I have.' That's what she had told me, and I prayed I would see her bouncing back before too long. Somehow, I had a feeling that she would. I think you can make your own luck in this world, and Mrs Sully had just the right nature to attract good fortune and be blessed with another chance.

Chapter Sixteen

'Your baby is showing signs of life
… He's alive!'

'So, Linda, which have been your most memorable births so far?' Marjorie asked as she coated herself in coconut oil on the beach.

It was July 1971 and Graham and I were on holiday in Marathon, Greece, with our good friends Marjorie and Colin. It was considered quite a luxury for ordinary, working people like us to holiday abroad in those days, and I felt very grateful for the break. I'd looked forward to it more each month as we put savings aside.

I'd been abroad with Sue to Beirut and Turkey, of course, and as a child I'd been to France, but I was thrilled to be taking a foreign holiday with Graham for the first time. Knowing I had such a treat to aim for had really helped me cope at work. I'd been busier than I ever could have imagined: after just six months working as a staff midwife, I had delivered more than 100 babies.

Marjorie never tired of asking about my work, and I was flattered by her interest. I welcomed the opportunity to tell her about some of my most interesting deliveries, as I'd been so rushed off my feet lately I'd had precious little time for reflection.

Unfortunately, Mrs Sully was the first patient I thought of because her loss was so recent, and still so raw in my mind.

Hers was just too tragic a story to share on this idyllic beach, though, even with a good friend like Marjorie. In any case I didn't imagine that was the type of thing she would want to hear about on holiday.

Instead, I relayed my favourite story of Geraldine Drew and how I'd got my wish and had the privilege of delivering one of her triplets earlier that year.

'I will simply never forget that lady, or the delivery,' I told Marjorie as I lay back in my denim-look bikini shorts and top, soaking up the sun's strong rays. 'She was such a character, and she was magnificent when she gave birth.'

I didn't share Geraldine's guilty secret, of course, as it wouldn't have been right to break that confidence, but still Marjorie was hanging on my every word.

'Midwifery is such a worthwhile job, and so interesting!' she said, eyes ablaze under the fiery sun. 'I bet you are constantly surprised, aren't you?'

'You could say that,' I smiled. 'I must admit I've had one or two women whisper to me in antenatal clinic, "I don't know if it's my hubby's. Can you work out my dates?" And one woman actually gave birth without telling her husband.'

'Never!' Marjorie exclaimed. 'How on earth did she manage that?'

'She was very smart and professional and always came to antenatal classes in her work suit, during her lunch break I assume. Her husband was away working on the oil rigs, that's what she told me. When he didn't even accompany her to the hospital when she gave birth I thought it was a bit strange, but I could never have predicted what would happen next.'

Marjorie was wide-eyed with anticipation. 'What did happen?'

'She had the baby adopted and went back to work the next day as if nothing ever happened. It's my guess she never told her husband a thing.'

Marjorie was fanning herself rapidly with a copy of *The Lady*. 'I'm blushing just thinking about that,' she said, adjusting the wide shoulder straps on her rather matronly floral-print swimming costume. 'How can anybody have the nerve to do that? And how can they live with themselves?'

She looked at me, as if expecting an answer.

'Don't ask me!' I retorted. 'It's certainly not my job to judge the patients. My job is to make each lady feel like the most important pregnant lady in the world, whatever her circumstances. And anyway, most women aren't so different. Pregnancy is a great equaliser.'

'I hadn't thought of it like that,' Marjorie said. 'You're wiser than your years, Linda Buckley! Tell me another story, go on!'

'Let me see,' I said, trawling my mind. 'This is another of my favourites. It happened about five months ago, when I was on nights.'

Our husbands appeared just at that moment, casting shadows over us and asking us if we wanted to book an excursion to visit the famous Parthenon temple in Athens.

'Hush!' Marjorie said impatiently. 'Just a minute! I'm listening to Linda.'

With such a captivated listener, I couldn't help but rise to the challenge. I settled into my sun-lounger and, whilst the men disappeared to have a cold beer, I told Marjorie all about Muriel Turner's delivery, in as much detail as I could.

As I spoke, the events of that fateful night came back to me so vividly I could have been on duty in hospital instead of lying on a beach. Muriel Turner's name appeared before my eyes as clearly as it had on that unforgettable night back in February when I'd been alarmed to see it on the admissions list with the words 'query, labour?' next to it. I'd seen Muriel at antenatal clinic the week before, and a quick mental calculation told me she was only twenty-six weeks pregnant. She certainly shouldn't be experiencing labour pains; it was three months too early for that.

'We've made her comfortable and told her to rest,' a pupil midwife told me. 'There's nothing else we can do about premature labour, is there?'

'Unfortunately not,' I replied. 'There's no miracle drug to stop the onset of labour, more's the pity. If she really is labouring all we can do is hope the bed rest will settle things down. I'll pop along and see her. Fingers crossed it's a false alarm.'

Muriel was lying very still on a bed next to the window, a terrified expression on her face. I had to walk past three heavily pregnant women to get to her, and Muriel's bump looked pitifully small in comparison to theirs.

I said a silent prayer in my head as I approached her. 'Please God, don't let this baby come now. It's far too soon.'

'Nurse, I really think it's coming. I'm sorry,' Muriel said. Her voice was trembling and she dissolved into tears.

'Now don't go getting upset,' I replied, wiping a tear from her cheek. 'Let me look and see what's happening.'

I drew the curtain around her bed and helped her remove her pants. As I did so she let out a whimper as a large contraction rippled across her stomach.

'It's hurting me,' she sobbed. 'It's making me push. I'm so sorry, I can't stop it …'

In the next breath Muriel pushed out the tiniest baby I had ever seen. Its skin was transparent, showing webs of veins beneath the surface. There was no sign of life, and its eyelids looked knitted shut.

It was a heartbreaking sight. Muriel said nothing, but just cried quietly. At twenty-six weeks, this would be classed as a miscarriage; technically she had delivered a foetus, not a baby. It wouldn't have been deemed viable until a fortnight later, when she was twenty-eight weeks pregnant. With such a premature delivery, we were not encouraged to attempt resuscitation unless there were signs of life.

I kept these thoughts to myself, not least because the scrap of human life before me looked very much more like a baby than a foetus, albeit a tiny, lifeless one.

I silently attended to the cord. The baby, a little boy, didn't breathe and showed no signs of life whatsoever. I laid his fragile body in a small green towel, which I placed gently in a kidney dish at the end of the bed before helping Muriel deliver the placenta.

Still I said nothing, knowing from experience it was best to wait for Muriel to ask questions, when she was as ready as she could be. Muriel was silent too, but the silence said it all. Her baby hadn't cried, and she knew what that meant.

I would take the tiny mite with me to the sluice for the time being, I thought, and clear up the equipment before coming back to talk to Muriel. I would have to place the baby in a special receptacle, clearly marked, and decide whether he should be sent to the morgue or to the histology department, for investigations. Head bowed, I carried the baby away in the kidney dish and placed him on the worktop opposite the sink while I cleaned the scissors I'd used to cut the cord.

As I switched off the tap and the sound of water rushing through pipes subsided, I thought I heard a faint little whimper coming from behind me. I span round on my heels, wondering if I was imagining it, but there it was again: the frail but unmistakable sound of the feeblest newborn cry I had ever heard.

I couldn't believe my ears. It was definitely coming from the kidney dish. It was Muriel's baby, letting me know he was alive!

I was up close now, holding my breath in shock as I marvelled at this little miracle. The green towel was moving. The baby's minute chest, just inches across, was clearly rising and falling; this child was certainly not giving up without a fight.

Clasping the dish tightly to my chest, I sprinted as fast as my legs would carry me to the Special Care Unit, which was thankfully on the same floor.

'Out of my way!' I cried as I ran down the middle of the corridor, forcing a nurse with a tea trolley and a lady in a wheelchair to swerve, grumbling, into the walls.

'What's up, Linda?' I heard another midwife call as I clattered through the doors of the Special Care Unit and practically threw myself and Muriel's baby at the nearest neonatal nurse.

'This baby is twenty-six weeks but showing signs of life!' I gasped. Though resuscitation was not routinely encouraged at this age, I knew help would be given in this instance, as the baby was clearly alive.

I handed over the kidney dish and said a little prayer to myself. 'Please let this one live. He's a fighter. Please let him win his fight.'

As the neonatal staff swung into action, allocating him an incubator and giving him oxygen, I slipped back to see Muriel, knowing her son was in the best place possible now. She was lying exactly in the same position as she had been before she'd given birth, very still and now with a devastated expression on her face.

'You don't need to say anything,' she said flatly as I approached her bedside.

'I think you might want to hear this,' I said, bending over and giving her a hug. 'Your baby is showing signs of life. I've taken him to Special Care. He's alive!'

Muriel's eyes filled with tears. 'Is he going to be all right?' she asked, incredulous. 'Is he going to make it?'

'It's very early days. I can't predict what will happen. All I know is he's one heck of a fighter. The nurses in Special Care are doing everything they possibly can to save him, and when I left him he was breathing.'

Huge tears dripped from Muriel's eyes and she shook her head from side to side, repeating: 'I just can't believe it! Is it true? I just can't believe it!'

I looked her in the eye and told her every word was true as I handed her a tissue. By now she had streaks of mascara running down her cheeks, and she was laughing and crying all at the same time.

Her one-pound, twelve-ounce baby boy did indeed survive, and Muriel herself was soon well enough to be discharged. I never saw her again, but while he was still in Special Care I kept tabs on her baby, who she called Liam because the name means 'strong-willed'. Little Liam stayed in hospital for twelve weeks, and every time I popped into Special Care to ask after him my heart was in my mouth.

'Slow but steady,' was always the response, thank goodness. He had lots of problems, some of them life-threatening. His lungs were so immature they collapsed several times, but I was very happy to end this story with the news that Liam eventually went home to his mum, and doctors did not expect him to have any serious long-term health problems.

'That baby was definitely meant to live,' Marjorie gasped when I'd finally finished talking.

I looked at her face, illuminated under the bright sun, and saw that she was grinning widely, yet had tears in her eyes, almost as Muriel had done in her hospital bed when she heard the good news.

'Look at you!' I smiled. 'We're all the same, us women. One way or another, childbirth makes you laugh or cry and quite often it does both – even when you're not the mother!'

We had a wonderful holiday, visiting all the local ruins, swimming in the sea and taking it in turns to launch ourselves off the diving board into the hotel pool. Graham and I had bought new clothes for the trip and I wore a beautiful long A-line evening dress with a silk choker collar for a special meal out on our last night. I felt fabulous.

'I don't want to go back to work!' Marjorie lamented as we shared a bottle of retsina at a local taverna.

'Nor do I,' the men groaned in unison.

All three looked at me expectantly.

'What?' I asked.

'Ready to go back to work?' they chimed.

'Actually, yes,' I replied. 'I've loved this holiday, but I absolutely love my job too.'

'That's it,' Marjorie said. 'I'm going to get out of that bank. I've made up my mind. I want to train as a midwife!'

I looked at her in alarm. 'You can't do that!' I said, worrying that I'd painted too rosy a picture.

'Yes I can!' she beamed. 'I'm going to make enquiries as soon as we get home.'

Marjorie was true to her word and did indeed set the wheels in motion for her rather dramatic career change as soon as we were back in Ashton. It would take her three years to train, but she was adamant she was going to make it. I am very pleased to say that Marjorie did eventually fulfil her ambition, and qualified as a midwife in 1975. She even worked in the new Ashton Maternity Unit for a while. I never worked along-side her, but by all accounts she made a good midwife. At the time, though, I must admit I wasn't sure it was the right move for her.

'It's quite different from banking,' I had cautioned several times on our return home. 'There are highs and lows like you could never imagine, often all on the same day. Honestly, it's like being on an emotional rollercoaster sometimes.'

'Bring it on!' Marjorie said.

One such rollercoaster of a shift happened in late August 1971.

'Come on girls, you can't sit down!' shouted Barry, who was one of my favourite ambulancemen.

From the nurses' kitchen I could see dawn was just about breaking outside. I'd been on my feet all night as we'd had a steady stream of deliveries throughout my shift and many of the women had arrived by ambulance. This was the first time in hours there had been a lull, and I was enjoying a well-earned cup of tea with a couple of staff nurses when the familiar sound of the ambulance siren wailed outside the open window.

'Come quick, Nurse!' Barry cried urgently, sticking his head round the door. 'Get off your backside! This lady's going to have her baby any minute!'

I rolled my eyes at him cheekily and stayed firmly put. 'That's what you said the last time, and the time before that,' I teased. 'And guess what? Those women are still on the labour ward despite their "emergency" ambulance dash.'

I drained my cup casually while Barry disappeared to help his colleague escort the patient, Mrs Cavendish, inside.

'The midwife's just coming, love,' I heard Barry reassure her loudly as he manoeuvred her out of the ambulance. 'You'll be fine now you're here.'

I headed down the corridor a minute or two later, and Barry informed me that Mrs Cavendish had been desperate for the toilet upon arrival and had insisted on being taken straight to the bathroom.

'That's good, I'll get her to do a urine sample while she's there,' I said, walking up to the door of the toilet next to the delivery room and giving it a tap.

'I'm not sure you've time for any of that,' Barry fretted. 'I told you, she's about to have the baby!'

'Oh, for goodness sake!' I chided. 'You ambulancemen are all the same. Always worrying the baby's going to pop out at record speed. It only happens like that in films, you know!'

'Mrs Cavendish!' I called through the door. 'It's the midwife here, Nurse Buckley. Can I trouble you to do a urine sample whilst you're in there?'

'Too late!' she panted.

'Oh, never mind,' I called back, thinking she'd have to drink some water and try to go to the toilet again in a bit.

'Come in quick!' she screamed, which took me by surprise.

Barry and I pushed the door open to find a startled Mrs Cavendish standing before us holding a grey plastic washing-up bowl containing what looked very much like a blood-smeared baby girl. Oh my word, it was a baby girl! The umbilical cord, still attached to the baby, was swinging between mother and daughter.

'Sorry,' Mrs Cavendish said, sounding forlorn. 'Found the bowl on the floor by the bath, seemed better than nothing. Lucky I didn't make it to the toilet, eh?'

Mercifully, the baby looked fine and began making a little grizzling noise as I took hold of the bowl with her still inside. I didn't want to lift her out because she was slippery and I was scared I might drop her on the bathroom floor. Mrs Cavendish, although clearly shaken, appeared to be in remarkably good form, considering what she'd just been through.

We needed to deliver the placenta, and I was very grateful when Mrs Cavendish agreed to walk cautiously to a bed just across the way, with me carrying the baby in the bowl on one side and Barry supporting her on the other.

Barry didn't say a word, and was kind enough to not to give me a 'told you so' look. He didn't need to. I was cross with myself for finishing that cup of tea and for being so cavalier. He knew me well enough to know I'd be mortified about it without any nudging from him.

Mrs Cavendish proved an extremely stoical patient and was on the postnatal ward with her daughter Hilary – her second child – within an hour of her arrival at the hospital. I went to see them before I finished my shift later that morning, still feeling deeply embarrassed that such a thing could have happened on my watch, and desperately hoping Mrs Cavendish wasn't feeling aggrieved now she'd had a few hours to gather her thoughts.

'Thanks very much for all your help, Nurse,' she said sincerely, stroking her daughter's soft head. 'I can't apologise enough for leaving things so late, but how lucky am I? I was in here labouring for twelve hours last time round with Hazel, my first one. Mind you, I think I gave that poor ambulance-man a shock!'

'Actually, I think you gave me more of a shock than him,' I said, truthfully.

I was very relieved that Mrs Cavendish wasn't complaining and, most importantly, that her daughter was not only unscathed by her unconventional birth but looked to be positively thriving.

Nevertheless, on my way home I silently scolded myself again for having been so arrogant. I was amazed at how cocky I'd become in such a short space of time, and I vowed never, ever to make the same mistake again. The ambulance-men generally treated us midwives like royalty, and from now on I was going to treat them with a lot more respect, too. Barry would no doubt give me some stick now the drama was over and no harm was done, but it would be a small price to pay for allowing complacency to creep in like that, and it would serve as a reminder to keep on my toes at all times, even when my feet were throbbing and my legs aching with tiredness.

Graham had bought me a little car by now and I was always particularly grateful for it after difficult shifts like that. Luckily, I passed my driving test first time despite making several mistakes. As my colleagues had cheekily advised, I wore my uniform and hitched my skirt up an inch or so, revealing far more of my black stockings than I normally did. During the test I hit the kerb while reversing round a corner, but the examiner simply gave me an admiring glance and said: 'I'll give you the benefit of the doubt.'

I was jubilant and thanked him profusely. Now I absolutely loved driving round in my navy-blue Austin 1100. It was a godsend to sink into the driver's seat after a hard night shift, and I wondered how I had ever managed on my moped, when my back ached and the early morning cold penetrated through my clothing.

'Nurse Buckley!' Miss Sefton bellowed one morning as I reported for duty and began unfastening my long navy-blue cape. 'Please report to my office in five minutes, and you might as well leave your cape on.'

My spine stiffened and I immediately wondered what I had done wrong. It was November 1971 now. Surely Mrs Cavendish hadn't complained about giving birth in a washing-up bowl after all this time? No patient had ever lodged a complaint about me, or any of my colleagues for that matter; it was simply unheard of. Nevertheless, Miss Sefton's brusque manner made that unwelcome thought enter my head.

I had been working as a staff midwife for eleven months now. By January 1972, after successfully completing my first twelve months, I had expected to automatically qualify for a sister's post. We would have finished moving into the brand new maternity unit by then. I had daydreamed many times about how wonderful it would be to work with all the new equipment and modern facilities.

Recently, we had benefited from a new centralised system of sterilisation in the old hospital. For midwives, this meant that, instead of having to sterilise instruments ourselves, all the equipment needed for a delivery arrived on the ward sterile and ready to use in a handy sealed pack. This was a huge help, and I could only imagine how much better life would become when we moved into the new unit. I'd heard rumours we would get luxuries such as disposable nappies and ready-made formula milk, and I thought how much easier it would be if sterilising bottles and preparing feeds became a thing of the past too.

Now, though, my hands were clammy and I wondered if I'd somehow jeopardised my chance of working in the new building. Whatever was the matter?

'We need to see Matron,' Miss Sefton announced stiffly, looking at her watch in an agitated fashion, when I reported to her office. 'Follow me!'

I very rarely saw Miss Ripley as she was usually in the Infirmary part of the hospital. Going to see her was a big deal. This must be something important, and I was seriously starting to panic. Miss Sefton was marching, sergeant major-like now, and I fell in line and followed her obediently, my heart pounding in my chest and my mouth paper dry.

We crossed the grounds at break-neck speed without talking, and Miss Sefton headed towards a heavy wooden door just inside the Infirmary. Pausing outside momentarily, she glanced at my worried face for the first time since I had arrived at her office and, surprisingly, gave me a reassuring smile.

'Don't fret, Nurse Buckley!' she said. 'You have done nothing wrong. Quite the contrary!'

With that she knocked briskly on the big door before pulling it open with a flourish and ushering me inside. To my amazement, projected on the wall opposite was a giant-sized picture of *me*, dressed in my nurse's uniform and holding a beautiful newborn baby wrapped in a blanket.

'Hello, Nurse Buckley!' Matron beamed enthusiastically. '*Thank you* for coming. We would like to ask if we may have your permission to use your photograph to advertise the new maternity unit.'

I was completely taken aback and wanted to cry with relief. 'Of course, Matron,' I stuttered. 'I'd be delighted.'

'That's good,' she replied warmly. 'I think your image is perfect for us. *Absolutely perfect*. Thank you very much indeed.'

A man stepped forward who I recognised as the photographer. 'Would you mind if we remove the little mole from your cheek, as in black and white it may look like a dirty mark?' he asked politely.

'Not at all,' I smiled, finally feeling myself relax enough to enjoy the moment. I felt the urge to jump up and down and clap and cheer, but of course I remained calm and demure in front of my superiors.

Weeks earlier two other midwives and I had been asked to pose for some photographs, each holding a newborn baby. The idea, it was explained, was that the best picture would be used on posters, leaflets and in newspaper advertisements to promote the new maternity unit all over the Ashton region, both to potential employees and to mothers-to-be.

The photographs were taken rather hastily after the three of us were herded into a single-bedded side room without warning, on the orders of Miss Sefton. In fact, the photo shoot had been arranged in such a rush that we had to run into the postnatal ward and ask some mothers if we could borrow their babies for a few minutes, to which they all readily agreed.

The photographer wanted an image that captured the look of a 'typical midwife', he said, and I didn't for one minute think my picture would be chosen. I was quite sure the other two girls were Miss Sefton's favourites, and I thought they were both far more photogenic than me, with naturally pretty faces and well-cut shiny hair. By contrast, my long hair was pinned back in a bun and draped across either side of my forehead like a pair of curtains. Scrubbed free of make-up, wearing no jewellery and with my nails cut short in line with the strict hospital rules, I looked decidedly plain.

I was photographed with several unsettled babies until I eventually found a contented little boy who didn't cry in my arms. I didn't know his name and didn't think to ask or look at his name tag, as I honestly didn't imagine our photograph would ever see the light of day. How wrong I was! That picture is now on the cover of this book, and I would dearly love to find out what became of my little co-star. Perhaps now I will?

I remember driving my mum all over town in my little Austin to admire the posters when they were pasted up on giant billboards and bus shelters in December 1971.

'Oooh Linda, look at you!' she beamed at every stop. 'Don't you look wonderful! Haven't you done well? Can we go and find another?'

She said the same thing each time we stopped at traffic lights and bus stops dotted far and wide within a thirty-mile radius of the hospital. Adverts eventually appeared in the local papers too, along with the slogan 'I'm crying out for you, Nurse', which was a call to recruit more midwives for the new unit. 'Any new hospital is only as successful and efficient as its staff, and so we're relying on you, the trained midwifery sisters, pupil midwives and staff midwives,' it said alongside my photograph, which was pasted in front of a picture of the new maternity unit.

Graham was chuffed to bits too. 'Successful and efficient, that's my Linda,' he chortled when he saw me smiling out of the pages of the *Ashton Reporter* as he ate his Rice Krispies one morning. 'I'm sure you'll have folk flocking to the new hospital after this.'

For me, this campaign was so much more than a publicity drive; it was an incredible personal endorsement. 'That's me, I *am* a midwife!' I marvelled each time I saw my own image smiling back at me as I drove through Stalybridge, Hyde or Droylsden. If Graham was with me I'd feign embarrassment, but the truth was I was thrilled to bits by those pictures. They made me feel I had arrived at last. I was recognised in the street and in the newsagent's once or twice, which also gave me a buzz, but the most memorable occasion was in the dead of night, when I delivered the first of several babies in the hospital car park. I will never forget the frantic young man who ran into the maternity unit, having left his labouring wife propped up against a wall, alone and in the freezing cold.

'Come quick, Nurse!' he shouted, charging onto the delivery ward. 'She's in the car park! She can't move!'

I had my head in some notes and when I looked up he appeared stunned. 'It's you!' he spluttered. 'Please come quick! My wife's having the baby in the car park!'

Mavis Crowther, a smashing auxiliary who was always extremely helpful to me, appeared at my side in a flash and offered to help. 'I've seen a few of these in my time,' she winked. I gratefully accepted her offer as I collected a pack of instruments, some towels and blankets and ran outside. Mavis, who was in her fifties and short and plump, grabbed her coat and scuttled along behind us as fast as her legs would carry her, clearly enjoying the excitement of it all.

We found the lady, Mrs Miller, bent over in agony and clawing at a wall in the car park with one hand while trying to hold the baby's head back with the other.

'The midwife's here!' the panic-stricken Mr Miller shouted to his wife as he sprinted towards her. 'It's the one ...'

'Aaaaarrrrgh!' came her reply. 'I'm gonna kill you, leavin' me out 'ere in the dark! Aaaaargh!'

'But you said you couldn't move,' Mr Miller argued. 'You said you couldn't take another step ...'

Wise old Mavis swooped in at this point and asked Mr Miller to remove his coat. 'We need to make a privacy screen for your wife,' she instructed, which made me smirk. I knew she was simply trying to distract him. It was 3 a.m., pitch black save for the glow of a nearby street lamp, and we were the only people in the car park. There was no need for a privacy guard, but it gave Mr Miller something to do to keep him quiet. Mavis also asked him to stuff a blanket down the front of his shirt, to warm it up ready to wrap the baby in.

I helped Mrs Miller out of her coat and, with Mavis's help, got her to lie down on it. She was clearly in a great deal of pain, but she was calmer now and did everything I asked her to do, even managing to joke: 'Mind me coat, it cost a bomb.' I could see the baby's head bulging through her knickers so I took out my scissors and cut her undergarments away. Moments later, a hearty cry cut through the damp and bitterly cold December air.

'It's a boy!' I declared. The baby had arrived so quickly there had been no rotation of the body, as would happen under normal circumstances. He was delivered completely in one mighty push, one of the fastest deliveries on my record. Mrs Miller burst into tears and her husband, still holding his coat aloft, sounded choked with emotion as he asked if the little mite was all right.

'He looks absolutely fine to me,' I said, cutting the cord swiftly with ice-cold fingers, and feeling very grateful we had

delivery packs at our disposal, with all the instruments sterilised and ready to use.

I knew we had to get this baby and mother inside in the
warm as quickly as possible. Labour and delivery may have
taken place in a sub-zero car park, but Mrs Miller would be
much more comfortable if stage three, the delivery of the
placenta, took place inside the hospital.

As I wrapped the baby in the blanket Mr Miller had warmed
inside his shirt, Mavis stepped forward, unbuttoned her coat
and popped the baby inside, snug against her chest. This left a
very relieved Mr Miller free to cuddle his wife while we
arranged to have a wheelchair brought out.

'Oh I do love kitchen midwifery,' Mavis chortled later,
when Mrs Miller was safely inside, the placenta cleanly delivered and her eight-pound son Keith was sleeping soundly in a
cot beside her. 'That was exciting, don't you think, Linda?'

Kitchen midwifery was a term I'd heard older colleagues
like Mavis use to describe deliveries that took place in unusual
or unexpected places, often without the correct equipment.

'Well, it was OK,' I said cautiously, thinking that exciting
wasn't quite the word I would use. Alarming and dramatic
were perhaps more apt. 'Mr and Mrs Miller will have a good
story to tell little Keith when he's older,' I added.

Mavis laughed. 'Yes, especially as they had the hospital's
most famous midwife deliver him!'

I'd been so focused on delivering this baby safely, I'd
completely forgotten Mr Miller's reaction when he first saw
me on the ward. He later explained to Mavis that he had seen
my poster smiling down from an advertising hoarding as he
waited impatiently at a set of red lights on the way to the
hospital.

'Fancy that,' Mavis chuckled. 'As if Mr Miller hadn't had enough surprises for one night without running into you as well!' Giving me a warm smile, she added, 'Lucky man, I reckon. You're a wonderful little midwife.'

Mavis's generous words meant a great deal to me. She was an auxiliary, not a nurse or midwife, but she had many years of experience under her belt and I valued her opinion enormously. Mavis was magic, and auxiliaries like her played a vital role in hospital life.

I went home later feeling on top of the world. I was twenty-three years old and, thanks to the posters, I was being publicly hailed as a fine example of a competent qualified nurse and midwife. What more could I wish for? Mavis's endorsement was the icing on the cake. Days like that completely validated all of my training, all of my hard work.

I thought about the homesickness, the worry, the blood, the sweat and all those tears I'd mopped up over the years, many of them my own. All of it, every hardship and hurdle I'd endured as a student nurse and pupil midwife, had been worthwhile.

I'd made it, and this midwife was here to stay.

Epilogue

The new maternity unit opened to patients on 4 December 1971. I wasn't on duty that day, but I remember feeling incredibly excited to be on the cusp of a new stage of my career. As I always do at times of change, I felt a little apprehensive too, thinking about stepping into this brand new environment. The unit had cost £2 million, and expectations were running high. As the poster girl I would have to set a particularly good example, and putting a foot wrong was simply not an option. I said a few prayers and unloaded some thoughts into a notebook to help prepare myself for my first shift there the following day.

This is what was going through my mind on the evening of 4 December 1971,while Mrs Kathleen Randle was making local history by giving birth to her nine-pound son Jarrod Matthew Rohan Randle, the first baby born at the new unit, at 6.25 p.m. that day.

Life is very good, but that makes me a bit nervous. I think Sister Mary Francis has a lot to answer for! 'You have to take the rough with the smooth, girls,' she used to say. I can hear her saying it, and so when things go well I always worry, just a little bit. Please God, help me be strong, come what may.

I have to pinch myself sometimes to believe I am actually delivering babies for a living!!! Graham and I are going to start 'trying' for a baby of our own next year. Fingers crossed for that. I don't think we'll have any problems. I can't believe I am going to be a sister very soon. Help me be the best I can. I know it will be really tough sometimes, but I can cope. I don't think anything can surprise me now! I want to always be a midwife, until I retire that is – not that I'm thinking of that just yet!

It makes me laugh out loud when I recall my words, because even today I still can't imagine retiring. I tried to leave Tameside Hospital, as Ashton General was later renamed, when I turned sixty in 2008, but I hated not working as a midwife and I lasted just three weeks before I asked for my job back and became a part-time community midwife.

So, the midwife is still here, more than four decades on and counting. I'm honoured to have become Tameside Hospital's longest-serving midwife, and to have been celebrated as one of the UK's longest-serving midwives as well. It's an achievement that makes me feel as proud as I did when I saw my twenty-three-year-old self smiling out of those posters back in 1971, but of course that's not my motivation for still doing the job.

I continue to serve the women of Tameside, some of whom I actually delivered many moons ago, because each and every birth still thrills me to the core. Feeling the warmth of a newborn baby in my hands is honestly as joyful and exhilarating today as when I nervously delivered my first baby, little Lorinda Louise Willis, back in September 1970.

It tickles me no end when I remember thinking to myself, 'I don't think anything can surprise me now!' You never *stop* being surprised when you are a midwife. The job takes you into the hearts and homes of so many wonderful and interesting women, at such a significant time in their life, that you never know what is in store.

Little did I know back then that I had over four decades of surprises ahead of me, some more heart-breaking than I could ever have imagined, others so touching, so funny or so uplifting they would take my breath way. There wasn't enough room for them in one book so I'm currently working on another.

My job has helped keep me going through heartbreaks of my own, and when I remember my youthful hope and expectation that Graham and I would not encounter any problems, I gasp at my naïvety. We did have the baby we longed for and our son Jonathan was born in 1974, but sadly Graham and I grew apart and separated when Jonathan was just a toddler.

I am sixty-four years old now and I know that only one thing in life is certain: babies keep coming, same as they always have, same as they always will. No mother on earth escapes without problems of one sort or another, whether they start at conception, birth or in the years of mothering that lie ahead. Why, then, do women keep having babies? It's a question I've been asked many, many times, typically between ear-splitting screams, in the throes of a painful labour! The answer, of course, is achingly simple. Babies are our lifeblood. They make this world of ours go round and round. Babies enthral and inspire us, giving meaning and purpose to our lives, whoever we are and whatever we believe. That is why I feel so very privileged to be a midwife, and why I continue to do the job I love.

No matter how many babies I deliver, each and every one is a miracle, connecting me to the world like nothing else, reminding me that we are all equal in the beginning, and in the end. It's a great leveller, childbirth.

Acknowledgements

It has been a life-affirming experience to write this book, and I am grateful to many old friends and colleagues who have helped me recall the past. Some memories have made me shake with laughter and cringe with embarrassment, while others have reopened painful wounds and brought tears to my eyes. All have reminded me how very powerful nature is, what an absolute miracle it is to give birth, and what a great privilege it is to be a midwife.

I would particularly like to thank the following people, who have all helped me to deliver this book, one way or another.

My son Jonathan, daughter Fiona and son-in-law Peter, who have always been there, telling me how proud they are that their mum is writing her story.

My brother John, himself a writer, telling me, 'Yes, you can do it.'

My friend Chris Pearce, also a midwife, who, when I doubted my memory, said, 'Yes, I was there and it really did happen like that!'

My colleagues at Tameside Hospital who have prompted my memory so many times.

The women of Tameside who have been in my care over the years, without whom my story could not be told.

Rachel Murphy, my ghostwriter, who is like one of my family now, and writes from inside my head.

Jonathan Conway, my literary agent, who would not take no for an answer.

Anna Valentine at HarperCollins, for having faith in me and for enjoying this book so much she has asked me to write another one.

To enable me to share my memories accurately without treading on anybody's toes or breaching confidentiality, I have disguised the exact dates of some births and changed the names of some former colleagues and patients, but by no means all.

The one and only Mrs Tattersall, for example, simply had to be identified and fêted as my inspirational community midwife mentor, as did Miss Bell, my astute Matron at the MRI, who somehow knew before I did that midwifery was the career for me. I am deeply indebted to both.